D1506629

CANADIAN MEDICAL ASSOCIATION

This book is endorsed by the Canadian Medical Association. The association's mission is to serve and unite the physicians of Canada and be the national advocate, in partnership with the people of Canada, for the highest standards of health and health care.

Medical Editor

Catherine Younger-Lewis, MD, MJ
CMA Publications

Advisors

John M. Dornan, MD, FRCPC
Assistant Professor of Medicine
Dalhousie University
Chief, Department of Internal Medicine
Saint John Regional Hospital
Saint John, New Brunswick

Erica Carson

Dominique Gendron, RD, CDE
Foustanellas Endocrinology and Diabetes Clinic
The Ottawa Hospital
Ottawa, Ontario

Phyllis J. Hierlihy, MD, FRCPC
Associate Professor, University of Ottawa
Division of Endocrinology and Metabolism
The Ottawa Hospital
Ottawa, Ontario

B. Anne Priestman, MD, FRCPC
Clinical Assistant Professor of Medicine
University of British Columbia
Director, Eagle Ridge Hospital Diabetes Teaching Centre
Fraser Health Authority
New Westminster, British Columbia

YOUR PERSONAL HEALTH SERIES

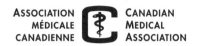

ASSOCIATION CANADIAN
MÉDICALE MEDICAL
CANADIENNE ASSOCIATION

# *Diabetes in Adults*

By Sara J. Meltzer, MD, FRCPC, FACP
and Anne B. Belton, RN, BA, CDE

KEY PORTER BOOKS

**Library and Archives Canada Cataloguing in Publication**

Meltzer, Sara
Diabetes in adults / Sara Meltzer, Anne Belton.

Includes index.
ISBN 978-1-55263-986-3

1. Diabetes—Popular works. I. Belton, Anne, 1946- II. Title.
RC660.4.M46 2009      616.4'62      C2007-904486-7

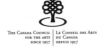 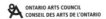

THE CANADA COUNCIL  LE CONSEIL DES ARTS
FOR THE ARTS  DU CANADA
SINCE 1957  DEPUIS 1957

ONTARIO ARTS COUNCIL
CONSEIL DES ARTS DE L'ONTARIO

The publisher gratefully acknowledges the support of the Canada Council for the Arts and the Ontario Arts Council for its publishing program. We acknowledge the support of the Government of Ontario through the Ontario Media Development Corporation's Ontario Book Initiative.

We acknowledge the financial support of the Government of Canada through the Book Publishing Industry Development Program (BPIDP) for our publishing activities.

Key Porter Books Limited
Six Adelaide Street East, Tenth Floor
Toronto, Ontario
Canada M5C 1H6

www.keyporter.com

Diagrams: Theresa Sakno
Editor: Paula Chabanais
Electronic formatting: Heidy Lawrance
WeMakeBooks.ca

Printed and bound in Canada

09 10 11 12 13 6 5 4 3 2

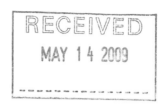
*To all the patients who have taught us*
*about diabetes and life ...*

# Contents

# *Acknowledgments*

We would like to thank all our colleagues and patients who, over the years, have taught us all we know about diabetes and living with the disease. In particular, thanks to the health care teams of the Metabolic Day Centre and Antenatal Clinic of the Royal Victoria Hospital with whom Dr. Meltzer has had the pleasure of learning and working for more than 25 years.

Also, many thanks to the teams at the William Osler Health Centre Diabetes Education Centres with whom Anne Belton has worked for many years. Special recognition goes to those who have given us comments and feedback on this manuscript: Hema Bhaskaran, Karie Quinn and Carrie Mintz. In addition, we would like to thank our families for their support and patience while we wrote this book.

# Introduction

*Michael's story*

Michael lifts a heavy lever and pulls hard. Something he has done at work every day. But lately Michael has realized he doesn't have the strength he used to have, and has been more tired than usual after work, going to bed earlier but then having to get up in the night to pass urine. He's always thirsty and has to carry water with him at work. His wife finally convinces Michael to see a doctor, something he has not done for years. The doctor explains that these are not symptoms of getting older but that he has diabetes.

You are probably reading this book because either you or someone close to you has developed diabetes mellitus. You may be feeling overwhelmed by the diagnosis. For most people the diagnosis is an unwelcome shock. However, some of you may have been expecting the diagnosis, perhaps because a family member has it or you might have suspected that you had diabetes but have delayed seeing your doctor.

Diabetes is not an unknown disease; you probably know friends, family or co-workers who have diabetes. In all likelihood, you have heard a lot about the disease, you know it means making changes to your comfortable lifestyle and you know it can have nasty complications in the long run. What you might not know is that the complications of diabetes can be delayed or even prevented. However, diabetes is not to be taken lightly. Those who live a healthy life with diabetes never take it for granted. They remain committed to their health and care of their diabetes as an important part of their life priorities.

This book is designed to help you live with diabetes, by helping you understand what diabetes is and how you can deal with it. The book is intended to help adults with diabetes. If you are parents of or caring for children with diabetes, refer to the publication in this series titled, *When Your Child Has Diabetes*. The diagnosis of diabetes and living with it raises many issues and will test your ability to cope. Most of you reading this book will have type 2 diabetes, but some may have type 1. Since the basic tenets of treatment are similar for both types, we believe this book will cover the major concerns that must be addressed.

The book provides insight into dealing with some of these issues and helps you, when working with your health care team, to develop a treatment plan that suits your lifestyle and allows you to live the best possible life with diabetes. From the start, it is important that you learn how to manage your diabetes and not allow diabetes to manage you. We have provided information related to the potential complications of diabetes, presented practical steps to prevent or delay their occurrence and, we hope, put them in perspective. The therapeutic directions of research, which hold hope for the future, are also addressed. Diabetes affects people of every ethnic origin, often occurring more in some groups—aboriginal people and people of Asian descent such as South-East Asians or Oriental populations. People of European background appear to have the lowest incidence of diabetes. Those treating diabetes must consider a person's cultural or dietary background. The size and scope of this book does not permit addressing details related to specific cultural or dietary needs. These are best addressed, whenever possible, on an individual basis with your diabetes health team, who are more likely to be able to adapt the basic concepts into your specific lifestyle. Your diabetes association may well have information specifically focused on your cultural heritage or even a local chapter or group.

This book is not a "textbook" of diabetes, nor does it attempt to cover every possible aspect of this complex disease. It refers and/or defers to other reference materials for more details when appropriate, functioning as a resource link to other useful information in print or on the Web.

## A Lot to Learn

At the time of your diagnosis of diabetes, there is a lot to learn. You will probably hear many suggestions for changes you could make to your daily activities in order to better manage your diabetes. Some of these recommendations will be appropriate; others might not be right for you. It is unrealistic to make all these changes right away—it takes time and lots of support from family, friends and the health care team. Your family doctor will tell you some of the basics at the time of diagnosis and then might refer you to a dietitian and a diabetes nurse educator or a diabetes education center. Your doctor might refer you to a diabetes specialist (usually an internist or an endocrinologist). Although it can take some time to get an appointment to see these people, it is important to attend and learn all you can about managing your diabetes. Other health care professionals who might assist you could be the pharmacist, a chiropodist/podiatrist (who takes care of people's feet), a psychologist or a social worker. Your local diabetes association may also offer help; in some areas there are local support groups for members with diabetes. It is important to be prepared to ask for help and support from the people around you. Trying to do it all yourself can be overwhelming.

## We Hope That This Book Will Help By:

1. Addressing the main issues of lifestyle, healthy eating and basic therapeutic options associated with the treatment of diabetes.
2. Providing answers to your most frequently asked questions.
3. Making information easy to understand and to find.
4. Presenting instructional tools for adjusting your management plan to deal with other illnesses, daily life and life's pressures.
5. Reflecting up-to-date medical information and best practices.

You could of course read the book from cover to cover, or it might be more useful to first read the areas that answer your immediate questions and concerns. We both believe that, although the diagnosis of diabetes represents a major hurdle in life, it is one that can be overcome with the help of knowledge and determination. The skills developed by caring for your diabetes often spill over to enhance your effectiveness in other aspects of your life.

The idea of writing a book about diabetes seemed presumptuous and would normally not have come to mind. However, in the summer of 2004, we were finishing the final edits on a manual used in a course for physicians and pharmacists, and thought there was a need for something similarly "user friendly" for people with diabetes. The idea would be to help adults affected by diabetes and their families manage the disease, allowing them to get the most out of their lives without sacrificing their health. We had both seen many, many people with every variation of diabetes in the more than 25 years we each have been in practice (Sara as an endocrinologist and Anne as a diabetes educator), and felt that such a book would be helpful. Within days of our discussion, an e-mail came from Key Porter asking whether we might write such a book! It was a sign that we couldn't ignore!

The information about diabetes changes fast. As we go to press, we hope that we have incorporated the most recent changes, but more may come quickly. We suggest that the best way to keep up to date is to watch diabetes associations' Web sites, such as www.diabetes.ca (Canada), www.diabetes.org (United States) or www.idf.org (International Diabetes Federation).

# O N E

## The "Normal Sugar System"

The body is an amazing set of systems—many of which are involved in "metabolism," which we have called the "normal sugar system." Once we eat food the digestive system starts processing and absorbing the nutrients from the mouth, the esophagus (swallowing tube), the stomach and the intestines. In the intestines the food is mixed with bile (from the liver) and enzymes (from the pancreas). Most nutrients are absorbed from the intestines and the remnants are excreted. The circulatory system delivers the nutrients to the body. The endocrine system releases hormones directly into the circulation to regulate the nutrient use. The renal system filters out the waste products. All of these systems are at work 24 hours a day to keep our bodies going.

*Joanne's story*
Joanne is a busy mom, getting up early to get lunches ready, waking her children, helping them dress and get off to school, walking the dog, heading to her own job, and working until 4:30 when she heads home. While her husband picks up

the children, she prepares supper. Once supper is over, she and her husband join forces to review the children's homework, clean up the dishes and talk about their day. She throws in a load of laundry and finally, after many hours of non-stop activity, falls into bed. Life is so busy—where does she get all that energy to keep going?

## How Do You Get Your Energy?

The first thing you do to get energy is to find a source of energy—you need to eat. The food you eat serves many purposes:

- provides you with energy for day-to-day activities;
- helps your body repair and maintain its parts; and
- maintains the hormone systems that keep your body running.

### The Major Components of Food

1. Carbohydrates are foods that are made up of natural sugars and provide the main source of energy for your body.

   - Some contain mainly sugars (glucose, fructose, lactose). These are found primarily in fruits, many vegetables and milk products.
   - Others contain mainly starches. These are found in grains, cereals or anything that you could make into flour or make out of flour.

2. Proteins are used primarily as building blocks to repair and remake enzymes and body parts.
3. Fats are used to make cell membranes, hormones and some other body systems. Fats are also an alternate source of energy.

**Carbohydrates** are broken down by digestion to form glucose. The glucose is absorbed into your blood and then moves from the smallest blood vessels, the capillaries, into your individual cells. The glucose does not simply flow into the cells. There must be a mechanism to bring the glucose into the cell—a "transport" system. This is where insulin comes in. Insulin is a hormone, a substance that acts to promote or change an activity in the body or a catalyst (something that makes change happen) for body processes. Insulin is one of the oldest hormones in the world, existing in the earliest and simplest of cells and organisms. One of the key roles of insulin is to stimulate the cells to put "receptors" on their surface to capture the glucose in the blood and bring it into the cell. It is only within the cells of your body that glucose turns into energy. Just as the individual cells in your body cannot live without oxygen, they cannot live without glucose. The energy produced in cells throughout your body helps you get through your day.

### How Insulin Helps Glucose into the Cell

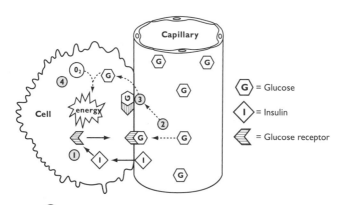

① Insulin enters the cell stimulating glucose receptors to go to the cell surface

② Glucose receptors connect with glucose in the blood

③ Glucose is brought into the cell

④ Glucose combines with oxygen to produce energy within the cell

Once the glucose is in the cell, insulin acts in many ways to maximize the cell's energy production, directing its activities to important cell functions.

- In the presence of extra glucose, as in a very big meal, insulin helps the liver and muscle store the extra glucose, mainly as glycogen, for later use.
- The ability of the cell to use proteins that remake parts of other cells or develop or repair special organs depends on the right amount of insulin being in the right place at the right time.
- The way the fat in your blood is managed requires an accurate amount of insulin. When you don't eat and your body switches to using fat as a source of fuel, insulin is essential to the process of allowing you to use those "free fatty acids" properly. If you eat a lot, insulin helps with storage of fat so it can be used later.

Even if you do not eat well or for some reason you cannot get food, your body will make some glucose by releasing stored substances, such as glycogen, or converting the fat in your body to a usable fuel called free fatty acids. Insulin is essential in these processes too.

Insulin is a crucial and very busy hormone!

## Where Does Insulin Come From?
Insulin is produced by specialized cells in an organ called the pancreas that lies just behind your stomach. The pancreas is part of the gastrointestinal system, the system that includes

your esophagus (swallowing tube), stomach (the "gastro" in gastrointestinal), the liver, the pancreas and the intestines. The major role of the pancreas is to provide you with enzymes that break down the food you eat and allow you to absorb it through your intestines. The pancreas is composed mainly of many cells that produce enzymes. The enzymes drain into a pancreatic duct that then empties into the very top of the intestines, just below the stomach. These enzymes help the body digest the foods you eat.

Sprinkled throughout the pancreatic duct system are a number of small collections of cells that produce hormones. These are called the "Islets of Langerhans." The islets are made up of the following types of cells:

- beta cells—the main group of cells that make insulin;
- alpha cells—a small numbers of cells that make another hormone called glucagon; and
- delta cells—very few cells that make a third hormone called somatostatin.

The islets have small capillary blood vessels all through them. The cells in the islets "read" the glucose level in your blood as it passes by and then respond by releasing the right amounts of insulin, glucagon or somatostatin directly into your blood. If the pancreas is removed or destroyed the body cannot use its glucose properly. Drs. Banting and Best removed the pancreata from dogs in their efforts to find and make insulin.

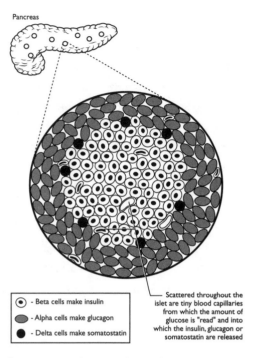

Pancreas

**The Cells of an Islet of Langerhans**

- Beta cells make insulin
- Alpha cells make glucagon
- Delta cells make somatostatin

Scattered throughout the islet are tiny blood capillaries from which the amount of glucose is "read" and into which the insulin, glucagon or somatostatin are released

When you eat food, your insulin is released in two waves or phases. The first phase releases insulin to help you use any glucose that is absorbed very quickly from your meal. The second phase or wave of insulin responds to the total amount of glucose in your blood from the meal you ate. This second phase of insulin release is slower, and adjusted to the needs from the glucose "load" in the meal. As the cells read higher levels of glucose in the blood, more insulin is released. After the meal, when the glucose level has fallen back to normal in the blood, the beta cells read the lower glucose level and turn down the amount of insulin released. This reduces the amount of glucose entering your cells and prevents the level of glucose in the blood from falling too low.

Joanne nibbles at her breakfast as she prepares lunches and gets the children off to school. Because she does not have diabetes, her pancreas gives her just enough insulin for the food that she is eating. Her blood glucose stays within the normal range. If she does not eat more, the glucose level might be at the lower end of normal and she might start to feel hungry; this would be a sign that her body needs glucose for fuel. However, her body will give her only the amount of insulin she needs for the food she has eaten, so she will not have a glucose level that is too low.

> **Metabolism** is the term used to describe the many different biochemical processes required for life (breakdown, re-building and adjusting) that occur constantly in your body. These processes play a major role in the digestion and processing of our food to produce energy.

## How Does the Body Ensure It Gets the Right Amount of Insulin?

If the body or beta cells overshoot and produce too much insulin, glucose may fall too low. Another hormone called glucagon would then be released to bring the glucose back to normal, at least for a short time. Glucagon works by telling the liver to release some of its stored glucose. The body has many mechanisms to adapt and adjust to its needs.

- In the gastrointestinal tract, hormones produced at various places in the stomach and intestines signal the body when food has arrived and also signal the brain when there is enough food and you should stop eating. The most important of these hormones is called GLP-1 (Glucagon-like protein-1). This hormone increases the ability of the islet cells to read and respond to the glucose in the meal. GLP-1 also blocks glucagon release after a meal. This prevents the liver from releasing extra glucose into the blood following a meal when you do not need

it. This hormone is deficient in some people with diabetes. (See Chapter 6 for more information.)

- The fat cells (or adipocytes) have long been thought to be
just an area where excess fuel is stored. We now know that
fat cells are important in the control of your sense of
appetite and feeling of fullness (satiety). We also know that
defects in the hormones that are known to come from the
adipocyte (such as leptin, adiponectin, resistin and others)
play an important role in the control of body weight.

- In times of stress it is essential that your brain and heart
muscle be supplied with energy to respond to any potential threat, either physical or mental. There are "stress
hormones" that work against the effects of insulin, dis-
couraging the glucose from going to less important cells
so that the brain and heart muscle cells will have more
glucose. The adrenal gland releases these hormones. The
hormones are called cortisone and epinephrine (or adrenalin). The higher the levels of these hormones, the more
resistant your body cells will be to the effect of insulin.

The cells of your brain and heart muscle do not depend on
insulin to get glucose to provide them with energy. They can
get glucose directly from the blood without insulin, which
means they always have access to glucose as a fuel. However,
such direct access also puts them at the mercy of the actual
blood glucose level that, if too high or too low, might affect
how well the brain or heart functions. In other words, they
may take in too much or too little glucose.

## What Is Insulin Resistance?
Resistance to the effects of insulin can occur in some people
with or without diabetes being present. When there is resis-

tance, the body increases the production of insulin to overcome the resistance and keep the blood glucose normal. If it fails to do this, diabetes occurs.

> When Joanne gets very stressed in her busy life, her stress hormones can help her body give her extra glucose to help deal with the stress. She may be temporarily resistant to insulin but, because she does not have diabetes, her beta cells are able to release enough extra insulin to allow the extra glucose to get into the cells and be utilized. Her blood glucose level will not change.

### Who Becomes Resistant to Insulin?

- If you gain weight, increasing the number or size of the fat cells, more insulin will need to be released to keep the glucose level normal.
- When a woman becomes pregnant, the growing placenta produces a hormone that counters the effect of insulin. Thus, all pregnant women make more insulin to keep the blood glucose normal, particularly in the second half of their pregnancies as the placenta grows.
- If you become ill or are on certain medications, such as cortisone, the stress hormones will induce resistance to insulin.
- In some families or genetic groups, there is a tendency toward becoming more resistant to insulin. Some of these genetically susceptible people have acanthosis nigricans. This is a condition where the skin on the back of the neck and under the arms thickens and becomes darker. This may or may not be associated with an increased tendency to have excess hair on the body (hirsutism), irregular menstrual periods in women or more little skin tags

around the neck. Those people, who have a genetic pre-disposition to insulin resistance, have a higher chance of developing diabetes one day.

Some people have a cluster of characteristics that are associated with metabolic abnormalities, such as:

- insulin resistance;
- elevated glucose levels, although not necessarily in the "diabetic" range;
- abnormal cholesterol or triglycerides (body fats in the blood);
- central obesity, that is fat in the abdominal area (the "beer belly" look);
- high blood pressure (hypertension);
- excess hair growth (hirsutism); and
- high uric acid.

This cluster of abnormalities has been termed the "metabolic syndrome." People with metabolic syndrome may not actually have diabetes yet, but are at very high risk of eventually developing type 2 diabetes. Efforts to improve the lifestyle of people in this group by encouraging healthy eating and increased physical activity may delay or prevent the onset of diabetes. There is often an association with "inflammatory" or reactive substances in the blood that likely plays a role in large vessel disease or the atherosclerotic process. In anyone with or without diabetes of any kind, the more metabolic syndrome abnormalities that are present, the higher the risk of large blood vessel diseases such as heart disease and strokes. Therefore, recognition of the metabolic syndrome provides a signal to you and your doctor that major efforts to control these abnormalities will help reduce your risks for cardiovascular events (see Chapter Nine).

Diagnostic criteria for the metabolic syndrome differ around the world. See the table below for the criteria used in North America and other areas of the world.

> For those with prediabetes (IGT or IFG) often in the presence of other features of the metabolic syndrome, efforts to improve lifestyle by healthy eating and increased physical activity may delay or prevent the onset of diabetes. In anyone with or without diabetes of any kind, the more metabolic syndrome abnormalities that are present, the higher the risk of large blood vessel diseases such as heart disease and strokes.

## Major Diagnostic Criteria for the Metabolic Syndrome

| North American Criteria National Cholesterol Education Program Adult Treatment Panel III (NCEP ATP III) | | International Diabetes Federation Criteria | |
|---|---|---|---|
| *Diagnosis is made when 3 or more of the following are present* | | *Diagnosis is made if central obesity is present plus 2 of the following* | |
| Central Obesity | Waist circumference > 102 cm (40.2") for men > 88 cm (34.5") for women | Central Obesity | Waist circumference* ≥ 94 cm (37") for European men ≥ 90 cm (35.4") for Asian men ≥ 80 cm (31.5") for European and Asian women |
| Triglycerides | ≥ 1.7 mmol/L (≥ 150 mg/dl) | Triglycerides | ≥ 1.7 mmol/L (≥ 150 mg/d) † |
| HDL | < 1.0 mmol/L (< 40 mg/dl) for men < 1.3 mmol/L (< 50 mg/dla) for women | HDL | <1.0 mmol/L (< 40 mg/dl) for men <1.3 mmol/L (< 50 mg/dl) for women † |
| Blood pressure | ≥ 130/85 | Blood pressure | ≥ 130/85 † |
| Fasting plasma glucose | ≥ 5.6 mmol/L (≥ 100 mg/dl) | Fasting plasma glucose | ≥ 5.6 mmol/L (≥ 100 mg/dl) † |

> means greater than; ≥ means greater than or equal to
< means less than; ≤ means less than or equal to
*Asian includes South Asian, Chinese and Japanese populations
mg/dl means milligrams per deciliter; mmol/L means millimoles per liter
† or receiving treatment

**What Is a Normal Blood Glucose Level?**
The body is amazing. Although you eat many different types of foods with varying amounts of nutrients in them, the level of glucose in the blood is kept tightly controlled. When you get up in the morning, your blood glucose level is between 3.1 and 5.5 mmol/L (55–100 mg/dl), averaging about 4 to 4.7 mmol/L (72–85 mg/dl). These levels may increase minimally as you age. After you eat, even a very big meal, the glucose level rarely rises above 7.8 mmol/L (140 mg/dl).

**How Do You Recognize Hunger?**
This may seem to be an obvious question, but the recognition of hunger is a relatively complex event, as is the realization that you have eaten enough. When you have not eaten for a number of hours, the level of insulin falls to minimal amounts and gradually your body starts to pull glucose from the stores in your liver and muscles. The changes in the levels of insulin, glucagon and other hormones signal the **appetite centers** in your brain. This produces messages in your brain that make you want to eat. When you eat, the ratios of hormones—such as insulin, glucagon and glucagon like protein-1 (GLP-1)—change. These changes provide feedback to specific centers, mainly in a part of the brain known as the **hypothalamus,** to tell you that you have eaten enough (**satiety centers**). However, this process is affected by the relative number of fat cells you have and the hormone levels they produce. The hormones from the fat cells, such as leptin and adiponectin, can affect the brain's response to the other hormones. The interplay of these hormone systems on the two major centers (appetite and satiety) in the brain affects how much you want to eat and when you want to stop. Stress hormones can affect this interplay as well. When some people are upset or depressed, they eat less; others eat more.

Many people have resistance to insulin prior to actually developing type 2 diabetes. Those who have developed insulin resistance may have similar resistance in their satiety centers, and thus may be less able to sense that they have eaten enough. Increased intake can lead to increased fat deposits that lead to more insulin resistance and even less ability to sense when they have eaten enough. This becomes a vicious circle that must be broken to effectively re-awaken the sense of satiety. Exercise, weight loss or an eating pattern that reduces the amount of insulin needed are all effective methods to reverse insulin resistance and allow people to again sense when they have eaten enough.

Overall, the body is an incredible machine, adapted to almost any situation that feast or famine can present. For the majority of people, it works incredibly well. For some, however, things go wrong, perhaps due to genetic makeup, environmental pressures (fast food, sedentary lifestyles) or simply aging. When things start to go wrong, diabetes can be one of the consequences.

# TWO

## Diabetes— What Is It?

The physician Hesy-Ra is believed to be the first to describe diabetes in the third Egyptian Dynasty. The description mentions polyuria or frequent urination as a symptom. Diabetes actually means "siphon or passing through." Mellitus means "honey." Together they mean "sugar that runs through"—the sugar is taken in and goes out without being used, which results in sweet urine. In fact, doctors used to taste the urine to make the diagnosis of diabetes. Even today, people are known to pour urine on the ground and watch to see if ants swarm to the puddle; if they do, the urine is sweet and the person knows his/her blood glucose is high.

Diabetes has not stopped people from leading full lives. Some names you will recognize are Bobby Clarke (National Hockey League player); Gary Hall Jr. (Olympic medalist in swimming); Halle Berry, Dale Evans and Carroll O'Connor (all actors); Ernest Hemingway, Mario Puzo (authors); and Eugene Ysaye (violinist).

There are different types of diabetes, but by far the most common is type 2 diabetes. Approximately 90 percent of people with diabetes have type 2; about 10 percent have type 1 diabetes. Some women get diabetes when they are pregnant. It goes away after the pregnancy and is called gestational diabetes. There are some rarer forms due to recognized gene defects or damage to the pancreas. Although the cause and type of diabetes may be different, the management principles are similar for all types of diabetes.

## How Common Is Diabetes?

Diabetes is a very common disease, affecting about 5 percent of the population in most countries. Almost everyone knows someone who has diabetes. Diabetes is found all around the world, but is more common in some areas. Curiously, people of European descent seem to have a slightly lower risk of developing diabetes. According to the International Diabetes Federation's Diabetes Atlas, India has the most people with diabetes, with about 46.5 million people in 2006; this number is expected to grow to 80.3 million by 2025. In fact, the number of people with diabetes is increasing worldwide; the World Health Organization reports the number of people with diabetes at 171 million in 2000 and predicts that by 2030 this number will at least have doubled.

### Who Gets Diabetes?

Diabetes does not discriminate; anyone can be affected. The number of people diagnosed with diabetes is only part of the whole. Almost as many again may have diabetes and don't know it. There are many reasons people may not yet be diagnosed—it could be that they do not recognize the symptoms of diabetes, they have not been to a doctor for years or there are no medical resources available to make the diagnosis.

### Can You "Catch" Diabetes?

Diabetes is not a disease that you "catch" from others like a cold or measles. The fact that it occurs in one person and not another is usually a combination of genetic luck as well as the lifestyle habits that people develop.

### What Is the Cost of Diabetes?

Diabetes is a cost not only to the people who have it and their families but also to society as a whole. When contemplating the concept of cost of diabetes, it is important to remember the costs are not only economic but social and human costs as well. Not only does the cost of diabetes affect the individual with the disease and their family, it impacts the society as a whole. In considering costs, it is important to remember, "an ounce of prevention is worth a pound of cure." The money and energy required to visit the health care team regularly, participate in regular physical activity, buy and prepare healthy foods, and the expense of preventive medications more than pays off over time. Since these expenses lead to less time missed from work, more "healthy" days and less "sick" days, and lower risks of any of the long-term complications, it is money and time well spent.

## Prediabetes

Prediabetes is a new term being used to describe people who have glucose levels higher than normal but not high enough to be diagnosed as diabetes. These people are at very high risk of developing diabetes and high risk of developing the macrovascular, or large blood vessel, diseases compared with a population not at risk of developing diabetes. This term has replaced "borderline diabetes" or a "touch of sugar."

The diagnosis of prediabetes helps us recognize who might benefit most from measures to prevent diabetes. Weight loss (about 5 percent of total body weight) in those who are overweight and regular physical activity have been shown to be effective in preventing or delaying the onset of diabetes in people with prediabetes by as much as 50 to 60 percent. Some medications such as acarbose, glitazones and metformin have also been shown to prevent diabetes in some people although not as well as weight loss and regular activity.

> Marc is busy with his university activities—his courses, the social side of things and especially with hockey, after he made the hockey team. But, in the last two to three weeks, he doesn't seem to have his usual stamina when he's playing. He tires faster than normal and he certainly can't party the night before anymore. He's also thirstier and hungrier than before, drinking soft drinks while he plays, which is something new. That makes him have to stop between periods and go to the washroom—his teammates are teasing him about that. He finally gets so tired he tells his coach that he's not sure he can go on the next road trip, he seems to get nauseated with the exertion in the game. His coach finally suggests he go to the campus medical clinic where a simple blood test explains it all. His glucose is at 25 mmol/L (450 mg/dl) ... he has diabetes.

## Type 1 Diabetes

In some people the onset of diabetes occurs quickly, due to an autoimmune process. These people have a genetic risk or susceptibility that activates their body's immune system when exposed to some trigger from the environment, such as a virus. The immune system gets the message that the cells that make insulin (the beta cells of the islets of Langerhans) are foreign tissue that must be fought off. The immune system then signals "killer" cells to destroy these "invaders" or "foreign cells," as if they were infecting agents or bad for the body. The problem is, these cells are essential—they make insulin. The loss of these cells by an autoimmune process can occur quite quickly, causing people with this type of diabetes to become very ill, very quickly. They cannot survive without replacing their lost insulin by injection. Type 1 diabetes usually happens in young people under the age of 35, but can occur at any age. The children of parents who have type 1 may inherit a genetic predisposition to type 1 diabetes. However, even if they do, they have only a small chance of actually developing the disease.

> *Pierre's story*
>
> Pierre has just come back from the doctor's office with the news that he has developed type 2 diabetes. He is very surprised at the diagnosis because, apart from being a little overweight, he thought he was in good health; he didn't feel any different. Although, on reflection, he realized he had been very tired after dinner during the past three months and finds he has to get up to urinate at least once or twice a night—something he never did before. Pierre's wife reminds him that his mother developed diabetes in her later years and that his sister had it when she was pregnant.

Many people with type 2 diabetes are not diagnosed early in the disease because they do not feel or recognize the signs and symptoms. See more about the signs and symptoms of diabetes in the next chapter.

## Type 2 Diabetes

Type 2 diabetes is usually a combination of two factors—insulin resistance and not enough insulin. Resistance to insulin might be a genetic trait and/or an acquired disorder. The acquired disorder can occur as early as in utero (while developing in the uterus).

Babies born with either very low or very high birth weights can, as adults, have relative insulin resistance and seem to be more at risk of getting diabetes. Studies show that as we gain weight there is a progressive resistance to the effect of insulin.

Activity also plays a role. When we are active, we need less insulin to move the glucose into the cells; if we are inactive, our chances of developing insulin resistance are higher. When the cells become resistant to insulin, the pancreas must make more insulin to compensate. Eventually the beta cells are unable to meet the increased need and become "exhausted." When the beta cells can no longer release enough insulin to maintain normal glucose levels in the blood, diabetes is the result.

Some other reasons a person might not be able to produce enough insulin include:

- A lower "reserve" of insulin means that when extra demands are placed on the beta cells it is more difficult for them to respond.
- The beta cells might have been damaged due to some toxin, so fewer beta cells remain.
- Consistently high levels of glucose might produce on-going damage to the beta cells.

In type 2 diabetes, there is usually a gradual decline in the ability to make insulin. Eventually, despite healthy eating and being active, most people with type 2 diabetes will need tablets and/or insulin to manage their disease.

We used to say that type 2 diabetes usually occurred in people over 40 years of age but the incidence in younger people has been growing in recent years, especially in some ethnic groups. This increase in the numbers of young people with diabetes may reflect the growing problem of obesity in today's youth. The relative roles of decreased activity and increased fat intake from

convenience foods has not been clearly delineated. Many community programs have already been successful in starting to
combat obesity by replacing fast foods with healthier choices
in schools. Some school boards have reintroduced physical
activity into the school day. There is a need for much more work
in this area of prevention.

## Gestational Diabetes

Gestational diabetes is a type of diabetes seen in 3 to 5 percent
of non-aboriginal pregnant women (up to 8 to 18 percent of
aboriginal pregnant women). During pregnancy the placenta
produces a hormone that makes the cells resistant to insulin.
Most women compensate for the resistance by producing more
insulin. Those who are unable to produce more develop gestational diabetes. Blood glucose levels usually return to normal
after the baby is born, and the woman no longer has diabetes.
However, she should be rechecked within six months after the
baby is born as she may have had unrecognized type 2 before
she was pregnant. She should continue to be checked yearly, as
up to 70 percent of women who had gestational diabetes will
develop type 2 in the next 20 years. This may depend on genetics and ethnicity as well as the lifestyle she adopts in the inter-
vening years.

## Other Less Common Causes of Diabetes

There are a number of causes for diabetes.

### Genetics

The results of genetic research show that there are many forms
of diabetes. Some of these include genetic abnormalities of:

- the insulin gene, so the insulin made is abnormal;
- the insulin "receptor" on the cell, so insulin is unable to work;
- specific molecules needed for the processes that insulin
  affects inside the cells, so insulin is unable to work; and

- the glucose sensor on the beta cell, so the cell does not release the insulin in the right way.

**Pancreatic islet cells destroyed**
- cancer
- pancreatitis
- some drugs for HIV/AIDS

**Drug interactions**
- corticosteroids
- diuretic medications
- some beta-blockers

**Other hormonal diseases**
- acromegaly or growth hormone excess
- Cushing's disease or cortisone excess
- uncontrolled hyperthyroidism

There are numerous rare syndromes, diseases, or abnormalities that are associated with diabetes. Additional information can be obtained about rare and unusual causes of diabetes in the Canadian Diabetes Association's Clinical Practice Guidelines published on the Web at www.diabetes.ca.

**Are Some People More Likely to Develop Type 2 Diabetes?**
The following factors are known to increase the risk of type 2 diabetes:

- first-degree relative with type 2 diabetes;
- ethnic backgrounds (South Asian, Aboriginal, Hispanic, Asian or African);
- history of impaired fasting glucose or impaired glucose tolerance, or gestational diabetes;
- presence of high blood pressure, abnormal blood fats, or known blood vessel diseases;
- very low or very high birth weight;
- age over 40;

- acanthosis nigricans—a thickening and darkening of the skin around the back of the neck and under the arms; and
- diseases associated with diabetes like schizophrenia or polycystic ovary disease.

### Do You Get Diabetes Because You Eat Too Much Sugar?

In the case of type 1 diabetes, the answer is definitely "no." The development of type 1 diabetes is almost always an autoimmune process that has nothing to do with your diet or anything you have done in the past.

In the case of type 2 diabetes the answer is yes and no. Some people have a genetic makeup that makes them unlikely to get diabetes. They could probably eat any amount of sugar any time they want and they would never get diabetes. However, many people have a genetic predisposition to diabetes, meaning a close relative has diabetes. When these people eat more calories than they need, they may gain weight that will increase their risk of developing diabetes.

Remember, as well, that most "sweets" or desserts also have extra fat content and significantly more calories than sugar-containing foods like fruits, vegetables, grains and cereals. These extra calories increase the chances of excess weight. Excess weight increases insulin resistance and therefore the chance of developing diabetes. As with anything, common sense and moderation is the key.

Diabetes is one of the oldest diseases known, with many different causes. It will manifest itself in many ways, depending on the person and type of diabetes. Whatever the cause and in whomever is affected, the basic requirement is to maximize the effectiveness of the insulin available to maintain the glucose balance and to let insulin do its myriad jobs.

THREE

# Diabetes—What Goes Wrong?

The major thing that goes wrong is that people do not have enough insulin for their needs. Without enough insulin, glucose cannot get into most of the body's cells, which leaves the majority of them starving for energy. Throughout this chapter we will follow the stories of Peter and Claire and how they came to be diagnosed with diabetes.

*Peter's story*
Peter is a 37-year-old schoolteacher who has an active grade 5 class. He has been teaching the same curriculum for years now, but this year, it seems to him he's not as energetic. He gets through his day, but when he gets home, he doesn't seem to want to play street hockey with his eight-year-old son or go to a movie with his wife. He feels tired .... maybe he's getting old. He feels like he's always hungry or thirsty or both. Over the last two months he has lost some weight, even though he is no more active and he seems to be eating at least as much as before. He doesn't sleep as well either; he always needs to get up in the

night to urinate. Lately he feels terrible, dizzy and nauseated, so he decides to go to the local emergency room.

### Claire's story
Claire has had recurrent vaginal infections that have been really irritating. She feels all right, although sometimes a bit tired, but then she is approaching 50. She is somewhat overweight and has high blood pressure. She has not been physically active since she went back to work three years ago. She decides to make an appointment with her family doctor to find out why she is getting the repeated infections.

## What Happens When There Is Not Enough Insulin?
There are both short-term and long-term consequences to insufficient levels of insulin.

### Short Term
Without enough insulin, the levels of glucose in the blood increase because the glucose is unable to enter the cells. The cells are then unable to make energy. Low insulin levels also have an effect in the liver. Insulin usually limits the release of glucose from the liver but when the levels of insulin are too low the liver will send out too much glucose, which still cannot move into the cells, because there is not enough insulin.

When the body's individual cells lack energy, the whole body will lack energy—you will feel tired. Tiredness is a symptom that people often explain away as not having had enough sleep, trying to do too much, not having enough fresh air or simply aging. Most people don't recognize the tiredness as a symptom of high blood glucose levels since it comes on gradually and becomes progressively worse.

Eventually, as your blood glucose builds up to levels that are too high, the body tries to get rid of it. Your blood circulates through and is "filtered" by your kidneys, which sieve out the things you do not need and keep in the things you do need. What you don't need is then passed out as urine. Usually the body pulls back all the glucose into the blood and there is none in the urine. However, if the amount of glucose in the blood being filtered is very high, some of the glucose escapes into the urine. All those extra particles of glucose moving into the urine pull water with them, causing excess water to be lost as urine— consequently, you urinate larger amounts more often. This can cause you to get up at night. The loss of water will make you thirsty, so there is a tendency to drink more water.

Meanwhile, back at the level of the cells, they are still not getting enough glucose, so they send out signals to the brain that they are hungry! Your brain senses hunger, often for sweet things because it senses a lack of glucose as a fuel. If you drink sweet drinks without any more insulin becoming available, everything simply gets worse. The higher the glucose level gets in the blood, the less effectively the insulin-making cells can work, so the whole process becomes a vicious cycle. You eat, but without insulin, the glucose circles around in the blood and some is lost by being passed in the urine.

When the insulin lack is extreme, more of the food that you eat "passes through" than stays. The cells have less and less access to glucose and more and more of the energy or calories from the food goes out in the urine, leading to weight loss. In those who have type 1 diabetes, this can happen very quickly, over days or weeks. In people with type 2 diabetes weight loss may be more gradual. If weight loss is occurring quickly for no apparent reason, the diabetes needs urgent treatment.

All of these events lead to the major symptoms of diabetes:

- fatigue;
- thirst;
- frequent urination;
- increased hunger; and
- weight loss if the insulin lack is significant.

Some cells, such as those in the lens of your eye, do not require insulin to get their glucose. The lens is a round, clear structure that light goes through. The lens focuses the patterns of light onto the retina at the back of the eye, which sends signals to your brain. This determines what you see. When the glucose level in the blood is too high, more glucose than normal enters these cells. This makes the thickness of the lens change, which changes the place on the retina where the image is focused. Your vision may become blurred when this happens, because your brain doesn't understand the signaled information. When your glucose levels return to normal it takes about six to eight weeks for the glucose to come out of the lens and your blurred vision to clear up.

In addition, when blood glucose levels are high, the cells that fight infection do not function properly, leading to frequent infections or infections that are harder to treat. See more on infections in Chapter Eight. The repairing of proteins that is needed for wounds to heal will also be slower because of the high glucose levels.

More symptoms of diabetes:

- blurred vision;
- recurrent infections (e.g. yeast vaginitis, boils); and
- slow healing.

Peter has type 1 diabetes. He felt fine until a few months ago but in the past two months he has lost weight and has no energy. He has no family history of diabetes. For some reason Peter's body has started an auto immune reaction and is destroying all his beta cells. He may have a few left at the time he is diagnosed but not enough to supply him with adequate insulin to meet his needs. Within five to ten years, he will be producing no insulin and there is currently nothing that can be done to stop that process. Peter needs to start taking insulin right away.

Claire thought she had no symptoms of diabetes but now realizes that the recurrent yeast infections over the past year may be a symptom related to diabetes. After all, she had gestational diabetes with her last pregnancy. She was not surprised when her doctor told her he wanted to do some tests.

## Long Term

Blood glucose that is above the normal range for a significant period results in changes to small proteins and the lining of your blood vessels. This can affect your eyes, kidneys, nerves and blood vessels all over your body, even in your heart, eventually resulting in the long-term complications of diabetes.

Your body also needs insulin to properly use and store the major fats in your blood, cholesterol and triglycerides. When there is not enough insulin, the amount of fat that stays in the blood will increase, instead of being transferred to the cells where fat is stored. If this condition persists, it results in a higher risk of changes to the blood vessels caused by too much or the wrong kind of fat. These changes, as well as changes in how your body deals with inflammation, increase the chances of macrovascular (large blood vessel) disease such as:

- high blood pressure or hypertension;
- early cardiac disease or strokes;
- abnormal circulation in the legs.

In the presence of extra glucose and not enough insulin, some of the glucose will attach itself to the various proteins in the body. As these "glycosylated" or "glucose-added" proteins increase, they tend to clog up arteries and change the functioning of some of the tissues throughout the body. The buildup over many years of these abnormal proteins can play a part in what is called microvascular (small vessel) complications. The small vessels can become blocked and the glycosylated products can change function, both of which can lead to changes in the eyes, kidneys and nerves, such as:

- eye disease that could lead to blindness (retinopathy);
- kidney changes that can lead to kidney failure (nephropathy);
- nerve changes that can lead to decreased sensation or pains (neuropathy).

There is more about long-term complications in Chapter Nine.

## How Is Diabetes Diagnosed?

Diabetes is always diagnosed by determining that blood glucose levels are higher than normal. This is done through blood tests. Fasting is just that: you will not have had any food for the eight hours prior to the test. Casual blood test is a blood test that is done at any time in the day. A glucose tolerance test involves drinking a specially prepared 75 g sugar drink and measuring the glucose in your blood before, sometimes at one, and always at two hours after to see if your body is producing enough insulin.

Diagnostic levels are as follows:

| |
|---|
| Fasting ≥ 7.0 mmol/L (126 mg/dl)<br>Or<br>Casual blood glucose ≥ 11.1 mmol/L (200 mg/dl) and symptoms of diabetes<br>Or<br>2-hour glucose level in a 75 g oral glucose tolerance test ≥ 11.1 mmol/L (200 mg/dl) |

Another blood test should be done on a second day to verify the result, unless the blood glucose is very high or the person is clearly ill. Blood glucose tests for diagnosis should be made at the laboratory—not on a home blood glucose meter. (There is more information on meters in Chapter Five.)

The values used for diagnosis of diabetes are based on the point at which glucose levels are felt to increase the risk of the complications of diabetes, primarily eye disease (or retinopathy).

Peter went to the emergency room and his casual blood glucose was 28.7 mmol/L (516 mg/dl). Peter has all the signs and symptoms of diabetes and was ill, so he did not have to have the blood test repeated on a second day. Diabetes was the only thing that could cause his blood glucose to be that high.

Claire had gone to the doctor for her routine annual checkup. Her fasting blood glucose was 8.2 mmol/L (148 mg/dl). She went back to the lab later that week for another test and the result was 7.3 mmol/L (131 mg/dl). Based on these two results the doctor was able to diagnose diabetes. Claire has decided to make some positive changes in her lifestyle and discusses with her doctor how she can manage her diabetes with diet and an exercise plan.

## How Is Prediabetes Diagnosed?

This state between normal blood glucose levels and diabetes has been called "prediabetes" because it often precedes the diagnosis of diabetes. Prediabetes is important to diagnose because there are steps that can be taken to reduce the elevated risk of developing diabetes and cardiovascular disease.

Prediabetes is defined as impaired fasting glucose (IFG) or impaired glucose tolerance (IGT) or both.

- In impaired fasting glucose your fasting glucose level would be between 6.1 and 6.9 mmol/L (110–124 mg/dl) and your glucose level two hours after a 75 g glucose drink would be below 7.8 mmol/L (140 mg/dl). In the United States, the levels for diagnosis of IFG have been set lower— between 5.6 and 6.9 mmol/L (100–124 mg/dl).
- In impaired glucose tolerance your fasting level would be under 6.1 mmol/L (110 mg/dl) and your glucose level two hours after a 75 g glucose drink would be between 7.8 and 11.0 mmol/L (140–200 mg/dl).

If you have blood glucose values in the prediabetes range, you should try to:

- Decrease your need for insulin with a healthy diet and an active lifestyle to prevent diabetes.
- Reduce any other cardiovascular risk factors, such as smoking, abnormal blood fat levels, and high blood pressure.

Although it is recognized that normal fasting glucose values do not exceed 5.5 mmol/L (100 mg/dl), the definition of impaired fasting glucose remains at values between 6.1 and 6.9 mmol/L (110–124 mg/dl). Independent of the level considered officially diagnostic, it is felt that cardiovascular risk may be increased at any level above normal.

## Diagnostic Glucose Levels for Diabetes and Prediabetes

| | | Fasting Blood Glucose | | Two-hour Glucose after a 75 g Glucose Drink |
|---|---|---|---|---|
| **Prediabetes** | Impaired Fasting Glucose (IFG) In the U.S. | 6.1–6.9 mmol/L (110–124 mg/dl) <br><br> 5.5–6.9 mmol/L (100–124 mg/dl) | | NA |
| | Impaired Glucose Tolerance (IGT) | < 6.1 mmol/L (110 mg/dl) | And | 7.8–11.0 mmol/L (140–198 mg/dl) |
| | IFG & IGT In the U.S. | 6.1–6.9 mmol/L (110–124 mg/dl) 5.5–6.9 mmol/L (100–124 mg/dl) | And | 7.8–11.0 mmol/L (140–198 mg/dl) |
| **Diabetes*** | | ≥ 7.0 mmol/L (126 mg/dl) | Or | ≥ 11.1 mmol/L (200 mg/dl)  OR Test anytime during the day ≥ 11.1 mmol/L + classic symptoms of diabetes |

*This test must be confirmed by another test done on a different day, either another fasting test, a random post-meal test or a two hour after the 75 gm glucose drink test unless the person is very ill. All tests should be performed in a laboratory, not done on a meter.

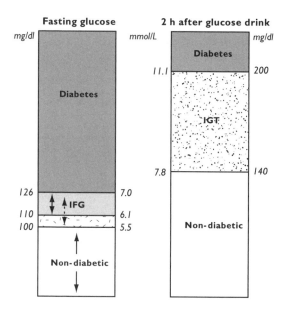

**Target Levels for Blood Glucose, Blood Pressure, and Lipid Levels in People with Diabetes**
As glucose is not the only factor leading to the major complications of diabetes, it is very important to address all the factors that can increase your risks of vascular disease. People with diabetes develop cardiovascular disease, on average, 10 years earlier than people without diabetes. So, if you have diabetes, a healthy lifestyle is even more important for you than for your friends who do not have diabetes!

**What Level of Blood Glucose Should I Aim For?**
Most countries have identified targets for blood glucose levels for before and after meals. The levels vary somewhat from country to country for various reasons that have to do with how the experts have interpreted the medical literature and how realistic it is to achieve targets in some countries. It is also important to note that target levels can vary for different people and at different times of life. Circumstances such as age, pregnancy, or illness may require altered targets. Remember that people without diabetes do not get the complications of diabetes, so the closer to normal glucose levels you can achieve safely and realistically, the better.

In Canada, the recommended target levels for most people with diabetes are:

- before meals— 4–7 mmol/L;
- two hours after meals—5–10 mmol/L.

Values of 5–8 mmol/L after the meal may be aimed for if the A1C remains more than 7 percent, always considering individual circumstances and the risks of hypoglycemia.

## What If The Glucose Value Is in a Different System?

In much of the world, as in Canada, the glucose values are reported as mmol/L. In the United States and parts of Europe, the glucose values are reported as mg/dl. It is not difficult to convert one to the other. To convert from mmol/L to mg/dl multiply the value in mmol/L by 18 to get mg/dl or divide the value in mg/dl by 18 to get mmol/L.

### Target Values for Glucose Control in Various Countries (Plasma Values)

| Country | Canada | United Kingdom | | United States | International Diabetes Federation (for type 2) |
|---|---|---|---|---|---|
| Pre-meal levels | For most people: 4.0–7.0 mmol/L (72–126 mg/dl) | Type 1 5.7–7.3 mmol/L (102–131 mg/dl) | Type 2 < 6.2 mmol/L (111 mg/dl) | 5–7.2 mmol/L (90–130 mg/dl) | < 6.0 mmol/L (108 mg/dl) |
| Two hour post meal | For most people: 5.0–10.0 mmol/L (90–180 mg/dl)* | 8.5–10.0 mmol/L (153–180 mg/dl) | < 8.4 mmol/L (151 mg/dl) | <10 mmol/L (180 mg/dl) | < 8.0 mmol/L (144 mg/dl) |
| A1C | < 7% | < 7.5%; if arterial risk, less | | < 7% | < than 6.5% |

* If A1C targets cannot be achieved with after-meal values of 5–10 mmol/L, a target of 5–8 mmol/L may be considered. These targets may be adjusted in special situations, such as for very young children, pregnant women and the elderly.

## What Is the A1C?

As mentioned earlier, some proteins in the body become "glycosylated" or have sugar added to their structure, in relation to the amount of glucose in the blood. One of the proteins that this happens to is the hemoglobin molecule in your red blood cells. Red blood cells live an average of 120 days and are constantly renewed. It is possible to take a sample of blood and measure the average amount of glucose that is stuck or "glycated" to the molecule of hemoglobin. This test is called the glycosylated hemoglobin, glycated hemoglobin, hemoglobin A1C (HbA1c), or simply A1C. This test reflects your average blood glucose level over the past two to three months. The result gives you and your health care team an overall picture of how you've been managing your diabetes.

The A1C is reported as a percentage—the percent of hemoglobin with extra glucose attached. There is a normal range, as everyone has glucose in their blood. Although laboratory reports may have different normal ranges, most often the range for A1C is 4 to 6 percent in people without diabetes. As seen in the table below, a value of 7 percent would mean that blood glucose values are averaging about 8.6 mmol/L with a range of 6.8–10.3 mmol/L (or 154 mg/dl with a range of 123–185 mg/dl), 8 percent would mean an average of 10.2 mmol/L (183 mg/dl) and so on.

## Glucose Levels Compared to A1C Levels

| Average Blood Sugar Compared to the A1C Value | | |
|---|---|---|
| Glucose (mmol/L) | A1C value | Glucose (mg/dl) |
| 16.5 | 12.0 % | 298 |
| 14.9 | 11.0 % | 269 |
| 13.4 | 10.0 % | 240 |
| 11.8 | 9.0 % | 212 |
| 10.2 | 8.0 % | 183 |
| 8.6 | 7.0 % | 154 |
| 7.0 | 6.0 % | 126 |
| 5.4 | 5.0 % | 97 |
| 3.4 | 4.0 % | 62 |

Rohlfing, *Diabetes Care* 31 no. 8 (2008): 1473–1478.

Most countries now recommend that people with diabetes try to keep their A1C at least below 7 percent, some as low as 6.5 percent. Lower levels of A1C have been shown to reduce the risk of complications from diabetes. One large study of people with type 2 diabetes in the United Kingdom showed that for every 1 percent decrease in A1C, the risk of microvascular complications (eye and kidney disease) decreased by 37 percent and the risk of myocardial infarction (heart attack) decreased by 14 percent.

---

The United Kingdom Prospective Diabetes Study began in the late 1970s and ran for more than 20 years. The study's purpose was to evaluate the progress of people with newly diagnosed diabetes. One group was given treatment to achieve lower blood glucose values than the usual recommendations at the time. The average age of the 5,102 participants was 56. The study was funded by the U.K. National Health Service. Further information can be obtained on the study Web site www.dtu.ox.ac.uk/index.php?maindoc=/ukpds/

---

## What Does Stress Do to Glucose Control

As mentioned earlier, those people who are more stressed will have an increase in adrenalin and cortisone, both of which will help them deal with physical and psychological stresses. These hormones are often termed "anti-insulin" hormones, since they interfere with the action of insulin inside the cell, resulting in higher glucose levels in the blood. This is usually protective, since it redirects energy to the brain and heart in emergency situations. If the stress persists for long or is chronic, these hormone elevations produce a persistent increased need for insulin that may not be easily met. Thus, glucose control might be worsened and/or insulin needs could be elevated.

Physical stress, such as an infection or elevated blood glucose can cause inflammation. The inflammatory processes might lead to noxious substances being produced. Studies suggest that some of these noxious substances might affect the process that thickens the lining of large blood vessel walls, increasing the chance for blockage of the vessels. Further information on this can be found in Chapter Eight.

### What Level of Blood Pressure Control Should I Try to Achieve?

Keeping blood pressure at normal levels has been shown to be very important in preventing the long-term complications of diabetes, and may even be as important as controlling blood glucose. Blood pressure is described as two numbers—the top number is the maximum amount of pressure the heart achieves when it contracts (the systolic) and the bottom number is the pressure in the circulation system when the heart is relaxed (the diastolic). High blood pressure causes the blood to put extra force on blood vessel walls, increasing the possibility of damage. Most countries now agree that people with diabetes should strive for blood pressure levels under 130/80. When blood pressure is higher than 130/80, you may have to take medication and, often, more than one type of medication will be required to keep your blood pressure within the normal range.

### What Levels of Blood Lipids Do I Need in My Blood to Avoid Blood Vessel Complications?

Lipid is a term that describes the various fat molecules in the blood. The best known of these is cholesterol, but triglycerides are also important. There are several types of cholesterol, but in this book we will describe only high-density lipoprotein (HDL) cholesterol and low-density lipoprotein (LDL) cholesterol. HDL is called "good" cholesterol because it carries cholesterol from the peripheral tissue back to the liver, helping to clear the body of excess fat in the blood. LDL is referred to as "bad" cholesterol because it is the smallest lipid component that carries cholesterol from the liver to the body tissues. Because it is so small, it is believed that it gets under the surface lining of blood vessels and this initiates the buildup of extra fat and by-products that might eventually block those blood vessels. The "total cholesterol" test result reflects all cholesterol types in the blood of which LDL is often the largest component. The ratio of total cholesterol to HDL is considered to reflect risk—the lower the better.

If your lipid levels, particularly the LDL, are out of the target range, you are at higher risk of macrovascular disease. People with both type 1 and type 2 diabetes can have lipid abnormalities, but they are most often associated with type 2 diabetes. A common pattern found in type 2 diabetes is elevated triglyceride levels and decreased HDL levels. This pattern can also be seen in the metabolic syndrome that can pre-date the onset of diabetes.

Physical activity, appropriate nutrition, and control of blood glucose levels are usually the first steps taken to address lipids that are out of target. Levels of triglycerides often improve as blood glucose levels improve as insulin affects the movement of triglyceride fats into the cells. Some aspects of the lipid profile are genetic, so they may not be modifiable. Whatever the reason for the abnormal lipids, if the lipid values do not reach target levels, medication is recommended.

In Canada, most people with diabetes should have an LDL-cholesterol equal to or less than 2.0 mmol/L and a ratio of total cholesterol to HDL that is less than 4. Other areas of the world have slightly different recommended target levels as can be seen in the table.

## Target Values for Lipid Levels in People with Diabetes

|  | Canada | United States | International Diabetes Federation (for type 2) |
|---|---|---|---|
| **LDL-C** | ≤ 2.0 mmol/L | < (1.8 mmol/L) 2.5 mmol/L | < 2.5 mmol/L (< 95 mg/dl) |
| **TC:HDL-C (ratio)** | < 4.0 |  |  |
| **HDL** |  | > (1.1 mmol/L) 40 mg/dl | > 1.0 mmol/L (39 mg/dl) |
| **Triglycerides** | < 1.5 mmol/L | > (1.7 mmol/L) 150 mg/dl | < 2.3 mmol/L (200 mg/dl) |

Claire's blood pressure has been ranging between 140/85 and 146/92 for the past six months. Her most recent LDL level is 3.4 mmol/L and her triglycerides are 2.3 mmol/L. Since her diagnosis, Claire has been walking 45 minutes every evening and she has been to see a registered dietitian. She states that her goal is to lose weight slowly over the next three months. The doctor decides to wait three months before starting medication to lower Claire's lipids. But the doctor tells Claire she should start medication to lower her blood pressure right away. If her lipids are still high in three months, she will then need medication to lower her lipid levels. If she succeeds in lowering her weight and exercising regularly, these medications might be decreased or stopped at a later date.

Diabetes represents a failure of the body to obtain appropriate energy from the food that you eat. Although insulin resistance is an important part of type 2 diabetes, diabetes will not occur unless there is a lack of insulin to meet the body's needs. Without insulin, energy is not produced and many other symptoms can develop. Management of diabetes is more than just concern about managing the blood glucose levels. Blood pressure and lipid management is of equal importance in maintaining good health and delaying or preventing the complications of diabetes.

# FOUR

# *Getting Your Head around the Diagnosis*

The diagnosis of diabetes might have been a shock. Or maybe it was expected; a couple of your family members have it and you knew it was just a matter of time. Perhaps it was a relief; you knew there was something wrong, you had been losing weight and feeling tired with no energy for some time. Thinking the worst, you were relieved when the diagnosis of diabetes was made. The initial reaction to the diagnosis of diabetes is different for everyone, regardless of how much you knew about the condition at the time of diagnosis.

People go through some well-defined stages when faced with any stress or trauma in their lives. The diagnosis of diabetes is a stressor and time is needed for adaptation. The diagnosis in one person will have an impact on the whole family, and everyone could experience the feelings discussed below.

However you might not all move through the stages at the same speed or even experience them in the same way. Be patient with each other—it does take time!

### Suzanne's story

Suzanne has just been diagnosed with diabetes and she is feeling overwhelmed. She just can't imagine how she will cope, she is angry that she has to make changes to her lifestyle, and she is fed up with people asking her how she is doing. She calls up her friend Marie who has had diabetes for many years. Marie listens to all Suzanne has to say and then tells her that what she is feeling is perfectly normal and that most people feel this way. Marie tells Suzanne that she needs to take it one step at a time and learn all she can; soon she will find she is living a healthier lifestyle than before and even feeling better!

On Suzanne's next visit to the diabetes center, she mentions to the nurse that she is feeling overwhelmed and a little frightened about diabetes. She is surprised at how understanding and willing to listen the nurse is. The nurse answers Suzanne's questions so that she is not as frightened. Then, together they decide that if Suzanne does not feel better in one month, the nurse will refer her to a social worker or psychologist who understands diabetes.

## Denial

At first you might have denied you had diabetes. Possibly you had no obvious symptoms; perhaps your elevated blood glucose was picked up on a routine blood test. Or perhaps you did have symptoms but as soon as the blood glucose dropped down and you felt better, you said, "OK, it's gone; it wasn't really diabetes." Or "The lab made a mistake; it wasn't my test that was positive." Because there might be minimal or no symptoms in type 2 diabetes and you may not have to take medication, it might be easy to deny that diabetes is present. Ignoring diabetes will have consequences, however, because the complications might be quietly progressing without your knowledge.

## Anger

Eventually, the daily activities required to treat your diabetes—planning meals, exercising, checking your blood glucose, taking insulin or tablets—make denial impossible. Now you might become angry that you have to fit all these extras into your life, angry that this has happened to you: "What have I done to deserve this?" "Why me?" "I don't have time for this." Being angry all the time is very stressful and can contribute to higher blood glucose levels. For many reasons, it is very important to move beyond the anger stage.

## Guilt and/or Bargaining

Anger often turns into guilt and/or bargaining, "I shouldn't have eaten so many sweets" "I shouldn't have quit the gym." Most people feel guilty that they have caused the diabetes. Even family members might feel guilty. "I didn't cook proper meals," "I encouraged eating out too often." Most of this guilt is ill founded. Diabetes is not caused by something you did wrong. Bargaining may or may not be realistic. "If I get back to the gym regularly, maybe it will go away." However, guilt and bargaining can be a helpful stage allowing you to re-evaluate your life and motivating you to get back into some form of exercise or start following a more healthy meal plan. As such, it can be a useful stage to move through, as long as it doesn't persist.

## Depression

After a time, you might feel sad about having to deal with all the demands and routines involved in dealing with and managing diabetes and feel that you don't want to continue this forever; you could be depressed. Depression has been shown to be about three times more likely to occur in people with diabetes than in the general population. Depression is also quite normal; your life as you knew it has changed, you need time to adjust. Watch for signs of depression; if they last more than a couple of weeks and are affecting your work and social life then you should seek help. Talk to your doctor or another member of your health care team about how you are feeling.

Symptoms of depression can include:

- loss of interest or enjoyment in nearly all your activities;
- either loss of appetite or significant increase in appetite;
- feeling sad, depressed, or discouraged all the time;
- either being unable to sleep or sleeping all the time;
- difficulty concentrating, perhaps finding yourself reading the same sentence over and over;
- difficulty making decisions;
- lack of energy or feeling tired all the time;
- thinking about death or suicide.

Depression is a normal part of the grieving process but should pass. If it persists or is severe it is better to seek help to resolve your feelings rather than to let them "brew" without resolution.

## Acceptance

It is hoped that you will come to the final stage—that of acceptance. Once you have sorted out this thing called diabetes, you will decide that it is not all that bad. In fact, you may be healthier having diabetes than you were before you had it—because now your blood glucose is improved and you are paying attention to your food intake and getting regular exercise.

You should not try to deal with the diagnosis of diabetes by yourself; talk to someone—a family member, a friend, or a health care professional—anyone who will listen. A person who cares will let you share your feelings without telling you how you should feel or what you should do. You need a good listener!

The more you know about diabetes, the less stressed you are likely to feel. Learn all you can from your doctor and the diabetes health team. Often it is possible to learn about the day-to-day realities and the emotions that go with them from others with diabetes. Look for support groups of others dealing with the diagnosis of diabetes. Support groups can be found at local diabetes organization, such as the Canadian Diabetes Association, Diabète Québec, the American Diabetes Association, or in association with a local diabetes education center.

## Managing Diabetes

There are many aspects to managing diabetes and although similar they do differ for the different types of diabetes.

In type 2 diabetes you may be able to achieve blood glucose levels within target range for many years by eating well planned and healthy meals, and doing 30 minutes or more of physical activity a day. Checking your own blood glucose is also an important thing you can do to help understand and manage your levels. However, you should know that in time, your body will produce less and less insulin, and you may need diabetes medication (either tablets or insulin) to keep the blood glucose levels within the target range. This is not a "failure" on your part; rather it is the natural progression of things, like getting wrinkles and grey hair.

In type 1 diabetes, you need insulin right away, but healthy eating is still a key factor in managing diabetes well and achieving blood glucose results within the target range. Physical activity also helps glucose and lipid control but the main benefit of physical activity in type 1 diabetes is improved cardiovascular fitness. Checking your own blood glucose is very important in helping understand and manage your diabetes. The lifestyle demands on someone with type 1 diabetes are often quite rigorous but, once achieved, can dramatically improve overall physical and emotional well-being. There will be moments when you want "time off"—unfortunately, it is not possible. You will learn to carry on, accepting blood glucose checking and insulin injections the way you accepted brushing your teeth ... a necessary part of your life.

## Making Changes

As you work through this book you will find areas of your life that you will want to change in order to better manage your diabetes. Changing the habits of a lifetime is not easy but there are steps that may make it easier, as outlined in the following paragraphs. There may also be times that you are having difficulty with habit changing. For instance, if you have not prepared well enough to make the change, it is less likely that you will be as able to sustain or keep to the change.

The first thing to do is to decide what you want to change. Do not try to make too many changes at the same time. Think about where you would like to start. Start with something you think will be easy to change, perhaps something you have been thinking about for a while. If you have success with one change, you will likely have more success changing other aspects of your life in the future. So start with a change at which you have the best chance of succeeding!

Making a list of the pros and cons for a new behavior often helps. Simply list the reasons this new behavior would be a good idea and the reasons you find it difficult or might not want to do it.

## Example of Pros and Cons for Walking Every Day

| Pros | Cons |
|---|---|
| I will feel better | It is too hot/cold |
| My glucose might be lower | My feet hurt |
| My blood pressure might be lower | I don't have time |
| I will build strength | It is not safe to walk in my neighborhood |
| My muscles will be firmer | I don't like to walk alone |
| I might lose weight | |
| My cardiovascular fitness will improve | |

Once you have your list, try to increase the pros. Then look at the cons and decide if there are any you could overcome. For instance, if it is too hot or cold outside, walk in a mall. Buy a good pair of walking shoes so your feet won't hurt. Find a friend to walk with so you can feel safer and encourage each other.

When your list of pros is equal to or greater than your list of cons you are probably ready to get started. You will need to determine a specific goal for this new behavior, one that you are sure you can reach. To set your goal, think about things you have done in the past—what did you enjoy? For instance, if your goal is around activity: what activities did you enjoy in the past? Can you do them again? What is your life like now? How can you fit in time for activity? Remember, it can be as simple as parking at the far end of the parking lot, or getting off the bus a stop earlier than usual, or walking up one flight and down two flights of stairs. If you walk for 10 minutes more in the morning, 10 minutes more at the end of the day and go for a 10–minute walk at lunchtime; that's 30 minutes!

---

### Remember the SMART Way to Set Goals
S   specific
M   measurable
A   action oriented
R   realistic
T   timely

---

### Set a Goal for Your New Behavior

Goals should be very *specific*; that means they should be only one action. For instance "exercise regularly" is far too broad a goal; "walk for 10 minutes" is specific.

Goals should be *measurable*; that is, you should be easily able to tell whether or not they have been accomplished. "Exercise regularly" might mean different things to different people. "Walk for 10 minutes" is measurable—you just need to look at your watch.

Behavioral goals should be *action oriented*. This means that to accomplish the goal, you actually have to do something, not just think about it or change your attitude or perception about something.

A *realistic* goal is one that you could actually accomplish. You would not set a goal of running a marathon in six months time if you have not even been walking daily. That would not be realistic. A more realistic goal would be walking 30 minutes for five days a week within three months.

*Timely* means setting a time by which you will start doing your new behavior, like starting the first of the month.

Example:
I will start walking 10 minutes after lunch every day starting next Monday.

Once you set your goal, prepare yourself to start. Do you need to get any equipment, such as a new pair of shoes? Do you need to get up earlier or leave the house earlier? Once you are ready to start, tell someone what you plan to do. Stating your intention to change increases the chance that you will actually do it. When possible, ask family members, partners, friends, or colleagues to be supportive as you try to improve your health by making changes to your lifestyle.

Once you have started, think about the things that might derail or prevent you meeting your goal. How will you overcome these potential obstacles—it might be the weekend, a vacation, or a couple of sick days—that interrupt your routine. Make a plan for how to get back on track.

Be sure to reward yourself for your accomplishments. Set a time for a reward—after one week, two weeks, or one month. Treat yourself to a movie or a new book or something else you enjoy. If you slip back into your old ways, don't get discouraged; think about the reason you reverted and try to avoid it in the future. Slipping back into old behaviors is very common. When it happens, try to remember the benefits you saw from your new behavior, build up that list of pros, and start again.

For most people the diagnosis of diabetes requires a number of changes to lifestyle, whether eating habits, activity or new behaviors, such as checking blood glucose. Remember, you cannot accomplish everything at once; setting realistic goals will help you to be successful and eventually help you to live a healthier life with diabetes.

## The Benefits of Diabetes

You may think it strange to talk about the benefits of diabetes! In fact, many people find that once they accept the diagnosis and make the necessary changes to their lifestyles, they feel much better and healthier. They have more energy and seem to get sick less often. And, if the whole family has embraced the changes, such as more physical activity and healthier eating, everyone benefits!

For some, the structure and discipline needed to keep a good glucose balance in diabetes will carry over into other aspects of their life—often to their advantage in succeeding in other areas as well. It all depends on how you "get your head around" the diagnosis!

# FIVE

## Lifestyle Adjustments to Diabetes

Everyone likes to eat! Whether you eat with friends or alone, mealtimes are a very important part of your day. Nutrition (what and when you eat) is very important for your overall health. The concept of a "diet" for most people suggests a controlled eating pattern for weight loss. However, the definition of diet is simply your pattern of eating. Meals that are balanced in nutrients and provide good nutrition will make you feel better, give you more energy, and help you maintain a healthy weight.

The way you eat is an essential aspect of treating diabetes. Balancing the food that you eat with the insulin that you have available is crucial. As this is not always easy to do, seeing a registered dietitian is helpful. We all have different body sizes, weights, and nutritional needs. Therefore, there is no such thing as a "diabetes diet" that is suitable for everyone. A registered dietitian can help you and your family develop meal planning and healthy lifestyle choices to match your needs. Registered dietitians are university-trained health care professionals who work in Diabetes Education Centres (DEC), hospitals, community health centers, and private practice. You may need a referral from your doctor to see one at the DEC, the hospital, or community health center, but there would probably not be a fee for attending. Ask your doctor or local health center about seeing a registered dietitian in your area.

## Goals of Good Nutrition
Healthy eating habits will:

- help you achieve target blood glucose and blood fat (lipid) levels;
- provide reasonable nutrient amounts or energy to assist you to gain, lose or maintain weight;
- improve your overall health;
- make you feel better and have more energy;
- allow you to eat your favorite dishes.

Yes, a healthy meal plan will allow you to eat your favorite dishes! Anything can be worked into a balanced diet; the key is to know what you are eating and how it will affect your blood glucose.

Important principles to consider when planning your meals:

**1. Eat a variety of foods at each meal.**
Food can be divided into four groups:
- grains and starches (foods made from flour or that can be made into flour like breads, pastas, potatoes, rice);
- vegetables and fruit;

- milk and alternatives such as yogurt and soy milk;
- meat and alternatives (meats, poultry, fish, cheese, eggs, legumes, tofu, and nuts).

A balanced meal is one that contains foods from at least three of the four food groups. Variety is important for both good nutrition and enjoyment. You should try to eat different foods from each group every day. That way, you will be sure to get enough of the essential nutrients, vitamins, and minerals in your diet. For example, potatoes, oatmeal, and rice are in the same food group but contain different nutrients.

---

### Be Sure Each of Your Meals Includes Three of the Four Following Food Groups

- Grains and starches (foods made from flour or that can be made into flour like breads, pastas, potatoes, rice)
- Vegetables and fruit
- Milk and alternatives such as yogurt and soy milk
- Meat and alternatives (meats, poultry, fish, cheese, eggs, legumes, tofu and nuts)

---

### 2. Space your meals and snacks through the day.

When you eat very little for most of the day and then have a big meal in the evening, you are asking your body to process a large amount of food and glucose all at once—it might have trouble doing this and your blood glucose may rise to unsafe levels. Glucose control is easier when meals are spaced out to about four to six hours apart. Some people find that smaller meals and snacks between meals result in better blood glucose values throughout the day. Depending on the type of medication you take, you might need to have a snack between meals.

Spacing your meals is important because there is a limited amount of insulin available. In type 1 diabetes, only the amount injected is available. In type 2 diabetes, the amount of available insulin is steadily decreasing over the years. When the meal has a lot of carbohydrate, you may not have enough insulin to ensure that the glucose moves into your cells. When the amount of available insulin matches the amount of carbohydrate in the meal, the resulting blood glucose after the meal will be within the target range.

**3. Increase the proportion of fruits and vegetables and whole-grain products in your meals.**
Foods are not all absorbed at the same rate; some take longer to break down in the stomach and intestines. This is good because it slows the absorption of the carbohydrate and therefore your blood glucose levels rise more slowly. Foods such as white bread will be absorbed faster than foods such as a bread containing seeds and whole grains. Fruit juice is absorbed faster than whole fruit. It is important to include starches with high fiber content, whole fruits, and raw vegetables in your meals.

Foods that are slow to be absorbed are said to have a low glycemic index. The glycemic index rates foods in relation to how quickly they are absorbed. Generally, foods high in fiber and less processed (for example, brown rice) have a lower glycemic index. The acidity of the food also decreases the glycemic index. This is why most fruits have a low to medium glycemic index. Try to include lower–glycemic index foods in your meals, or at least to combine low–glycemic index foods at times when you eat other higher–glycemic index foods. You can find lists of low-glycemic foods and additional information on the Web sites for the Canadian Diabetes Association, the American Diabetes

Association, or the international glycemic index site
(www.diabetes.ca, www.glycemicindex.com or
www.diabetes.org).

---

**Examples of Foods with a Low Glycemic Index**

Some bran cereals, old-fashioned oatmeal, natural muesli, apples, cherries, grapefruit, prunes, barley crackers, spaghetti, milk, yogurt, all beans, pumpernickel bread, sourdough bread.

---

### 4. Choose lower-fat foods.

Fats contain nutrients essential for your good health and fat in a meal will not directly affect your blood glucose level. The presence of fat will slow the digestive process, so a higher-fat meal will result in a slower rise in glucose after the meal. Although a slower rise in blood glucose can be helpful, fats are high in calories.

Some fats are good for you, such as the monounsaturated fats (for example, olive and canola oils). Other fats can produce negative effects on your body, such as "saturated fats" or "trans fats." Generally, fats that are solid at room temperature are saturated. Saturated fat is found in animal products or in foods made with hydrogenated fat. Trans fats are unnatural fats used to prolong the shelf life of foods. Some foods that contain trans fats are hydrogenated margarine and some crackers, pre-packaged snacks, and fast foods (a quick look at the labels indicates which foods have trans fats).

Energy from the fat in your diet should make up less than 35 percent of total calories, and of that, less than 7 percent should be saturated and minimal trans fats. Small amounts of fat provide high calories, making fat a source of concentrated energy. A diet high in fat will provide a lot of calories and may make it difficult to control your weight. You can lower your fat intake and improve the kinds of fat you use by:

- reading the Nutrition Facts on the labels on food products and choosing the products that have the lower level (learn how to read labels later in this chapter);
- buying lean meats;
- trimming all visible fat from meat and removing the skin from chicken before cooking;
- switching to lower-fat milk and dairy products. For instance, if you currently drink 2 percent milk, switch to 1 percent or skim and choose low-fat cheese (less than 15 to 20 percent milk fat).

Many of us eat more saturated fat than is healthy for us. Excessive fat intake, particularly unhealthy fats, can increase the chances of developing atherosclerosis (blocked arteries) and heart disease.

## 5. Limit salt and alcohol.

Salt does not affect your blood glucose but may cause other health problems. Excess salt over time increases the chances of high blood pressure and causes you to retain fluid. If you have high blood pressure, it is wise to use minimal salt in cooking, not add salt at the table, and limit the amount of salted snacks and processed foods that you eat. This often means limiting seasonings such as garlic salt or onion salt. Instead use fresh garlic, garlic powder, fresh onions, herbs, spices, lemon, and flavored vinegars to add zest to your food. With time, your taste for salt will decrease.

Most health guidelines recommend limiting alcohol to a

maximum of one to two drinks a day or fewer than fourteen drinks a week for men and nine drinks a week for women. Spirits and dry wines do not contain carbohydrates but contain a lot of calories and can make weight control more difficult. Beers and sweet wines contain carbohydrates and may affect your blood glucose. See Chapter Eight for more details on alcohol.

## Planning Your Meals

An initial assessment by your dietitian will help you determine the energy needs that you have either to gain, maintain, or lose weight. This is usually determined using a unit of energy measure called a calorie or a kilocalorie (kcal). The common term is calories, which actually refers to a unit of energy measure —the kilocalorie. To lose a pound of weight, for example, you would need to create a deficit of about 3,500 kilocalories. If you wanted to lose that in a week, you would need to eat about 500 kilocalories fewer per day. If that decrease in food seems too restrictive but you still want to lose the pound, it would mean that perhaps you eat only 250 fewer kilocalories a day and try to "spend" the extra 250 kilocalories per day by increasing your activities. Although calories are useful as a global concept, in planning your meal plan for diabetes management, your dietitian is more likely to concentrate on the balance of the meals and the carbohydrates that you will eat.

Carbohydrates are essential and form the basis of your meal plan, representing about 50 percent of the calories you need. Some people think that if you have diabetes you should avoid eating carbohydrates. That is not true because they are your major source of energy and contain nutrients essential to your diet. Each gram of carbohydrate contains only 4 kilocalories so a standard 15 gram portion of carbohydrate is only 60 kilocalories—that is less than 1 tablespoon of oil.

## The Plate Method

An easy way to plan your meals is called the plate method and it is used all over the world to help people visualize a healthy meal.

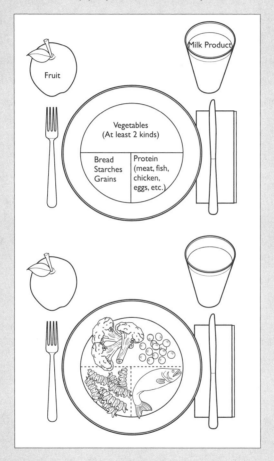

Half of the plate should be covered with vegetables, preferably two different kinds. One quarter of the plate should be grains and starchy foods such as rice, potatoes, or pasta. Some vegetables that are high in carbohydrates, such as parsnips, peas, rutabagas (turnips), and squash, should be counted as starches when in quantities of more and half a cup. The remaining quarter of the plate should be meats and alternatives, such as chicken, beans, or legumes. A glass of milk or milk alternative and a fruit finish off the meal.

*George's story*

George has type 2 diabetes, and he likes to eat! He usually does not eat much breakfast—maybe a cup of coffee and a muffin on the way to work. He buys his lunch from the snack wagon at work, usually a bag of chips, a sandwich, and a soft drink. When he gets home he has his main meal of the day—after all, he has been working hard all day and he is hungry!

After George was diagnosed and had read some of the information the doctor gave him, he realized he should make some changes to his eating pattern. He decided to change his lunch first because he thought that might be easier for him than changing his breakfast.

George decided to try to use the plate method for his lunch meal from the truck. He ordered a salad, a meat sandwich, and a fruit yogurt. He still likes his soft drink, but switched to a diet soft drink. He usually bought an apple from the snack wagon and tried to remember to eat it in the afternoon. He found that when he did eat it, he was less hungry for supper.

**What Is a Serving Size?**

The next question is how much of each of these groups you should put on the plate. Again, there is a simple way to judge amounts. This method uses your hands as a measuring guide and has been called the Handy Portion Guide. (Used with permission from the Canadian Diabetes Association © 2005.) It was first developed in Zimbabwe and has been known internationally as the "Zimbabwe Hand Jive" for many years. Those of you who are very active may need to increase or adapt the portions to your needs, ideally with the help of a dietitian.

One clenched fist is the amount of grains and starches on your plate. Your portion of fruit should be the size of one fist.

For instance the amount of rice on your plate could be equal to one fist, and a medium apple would finish off the meal.

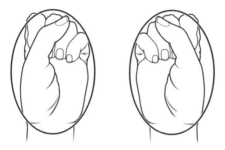

Most vegetables are low in carbohydrates and you can have as much as you can hold in two open hands. For instance, you could have a handful of broccoli and a handful of salad.

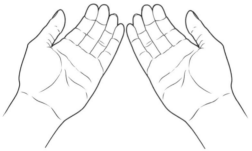

The protein or meat serving should be the size of the palm of your hand—that does not include your fingers—and about the thickness of your baby finger. For most of us that is not a 10-ounce (300 g) steak!

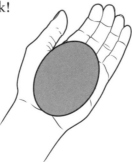

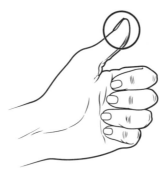

You can use a little fat (for example, a little butter or margarine on your vegetables or salad oil on your salad). The amount should be no bigger than the tip of your thumb.

A serving of milk at any one meal should be limited to 8 ounces (250 mL).

### Counting Carbohydrates

Another way to estimate portion sizes is to total the carbohydrates in each meal. Three of the food groups affect blood glucose: grains and starches, fruits, and milk and alternatives. There is also another group called "other choices" with foods like snack foods. To help you count your total carbohydrates you can use the carb choices system. Every carb choice contains about 15 grams of carbohydrate. For example, 15 grams represents 3 teaspoons of sugar because there are 5 grams of carbohydrate in one teaspoon of sugar.

The following chart shows sample serving sizes of foods and their carbohydrate values. For a listing of more foods go to www.hc-sc.gc.ca then go to Food and Nutrition and follow the links. Your dietitian is likely the best person to provide you with materials related to carbohydrate counting. When you know what a serving size is and how
many carbs you should have at a meal then you can select your meals by adding up the carbs. Let's see how this works.

## Fifteen-gram Carbohydrate Portions

**Grains and Starches**
1 slice of bread
1/3 cup cooked rice (not packed!)
6" pita bread
1/2 medium potato
1/2 cup unsweetened cold or 3/4 cup cooked cereal

**Fruits**
1 medium apple
1/2 cup unsweetened juice
1 small banana (or 1/2 large one)
1 medium pear
15 grapes
2 cups whole strawberries

**Milk and alternatives**
1 cup of milk
3/4 cup plain yogurt

**Other choices**
1 tbsp jam or jelly
3 tsp sugar, honey, syrup

Canadian Diabetes Association, 2006. "Beyond the Basiscs."

## How Many Carbs Do You Need?

Individuals need different amounts of carbohydrate. The amount of carbs you require depends on your age, sex, physical activity level, and your weight goal. The best way to find out what you need is to see a dietitian who will work it out specifically for you. Below are some sample meals with variable carb levels to help you get a sense of how it works:

## Sample Breakfasts

| | | | |
|---|---|---|---|
| I medium orange | 15 g | 2 slices French toast (made with milk and egg) | 30 g |
| I slice whole wheat toast | 15 g | | |
| I tbsp peanut butter or | | I peach or 2 kiwis | 15 g |
| I egg | 0 g | 1/2 cup fruit yogurt (no added sugar) topping on toast | 7 g |
| I tsp butter or margarine | 0 g | 1/2 cup milk in café au lait | 7 g |
| I cup milk | 15 g | | |
| Tea or coffee | 0 g | | |
| **Total** | **45 g** | **Total** | **59 g** |

## Sample Lunches

| | | | |
|---|---|---|---|
| Ham sandwich | 30 g | I cup lentil soup | 15 g |
| Butter (small amount) | 0 g | Chef's salad with potato | ~5 g |
| or mayonnaise and mustard | 0 g | 6 Melba toast or I small bun | 15 g |
| I cup I % milk | 15 g | 3/4 cup (6 oz) fruit yogurt (no added sugar) | 10 g |
| I medium apple | 15 g | Salad oil | 0 g |
| **Total** | **60 g** | **Total** | **45 g** |

## Sample Suppers

| | | | |
|---|---|---|---|
| I medium baked potato | 30 g | I cup cooked spaghetti | 30 g |
| 1/2–I cup broccoli | 0 g | I cup spaghetti sauce with | |
| I chicken breast, grilled | 0 g | onions, tomatoes, carrot | 15 g |
| 3/4 cup low-fat plain yogurt with garlic/ginger as sauce | 15 g | I small piece of garlic bread | 15 g |
| 1/2 cup vanilla ice cream | 15 g | Salad (green) | 0 g |
| 1/2 cup blueberries | 7 g | 1/2 cup grapes | 15 g |
| Tea or coffee | 0g | Tea or coffee | 0 g |
| **Total** | **67 g** | **Total** | **75 g** |

One of the advantages of counting carbs is that you can try a variety of foods and still stay within the recommended amount. Mixed foods, such as stews and casseroles, can be calculated by working out the total of the ingredients then dividing by the number of servings in the complete dish. There are many cookbooks available that have worked out the amount of carbs for you, or you may want to speak to a dietitian about how to do it.

Sounds complicated? Well it probably is a little complicated to start with, but give it a try and with some practice you will be counting carbs in no time!

### What about Fats?

Fats are important because they:

- are an alternate source of fuel;
- help you absorb vitamins;
- improve the flavor of food;
- help you feel full after eating;
- are necessary for your cells and hormones.

You need fats in your daily food intake but you should be careful about the amount and kind of fat. There are different kinds of fat; some pose a risk for heart disease and some actually help to prevent heart disease. The total recommended amount of fat intake is less than 35 percent of your daily calories. The amount of fat in a product is usually counted in grams, with 1 gram of fat being equal to 9 kilocalories. Currently the recommendation is that total fat intake should not contain more than 7 percent saturated fat and as little trans fat as possible. If you want to get a sense of what this number is for you, multiply the grams of saturated fat you eat per day by 9 to get the calories. That number should be less than 7 percent of your total recommended intake of calories. (See also Appendix One.)

| Good Fat | | Not-So-Good Fat | |
| --- | --- | --- | --- |
| **Monounsaturated fats** | | **Saturated fats** | |
| *What it does* | *Source* | *What it does* | *Source* |
| Lowers total cholesterol levels but not HDL (the "good" cholesterol) | Canola oil, olive oil, peanuts, peanut oil, and avocados | Raise the total cholesterol and LDL (the "bad" cholesterol) and increase the risk of heart disease. | Animal products and some oils, specifically palm, coconut and hydrogenated margarine |
| **Polyunsaturated fat: Omega-6** | | **Trans fat** | |
| *What it does* | *Source* | *What it does* | *Source* |
| Reduces overall cholesterol levels and may lower or raise HDL (the "good" cholesterol) | Vegetable oils such as corn, safflower, sunflower oil, soybean oil, and walnuts | Raises LDL cholesterol and decreases HDL | Formed when vegetable oil goes through a process that makes it solid— found in commercially bought cookies, cakes, etc. |
| **Omega-3 fatty acid** | | | |
| *What it does* | *Source* | | |
| Helps reduce blood pressure and protects against formation of blood clots | Some fish such as salmon, tuna, mackerel, and rainbow trout, and walnuts and flax. | | |

Your daily intake should have more monounsaturated and omega-3 fatty acids than any other kind of fat. The omega-3 and omega-6 fats are called "essential" fats, which are essential to normal functioning of your body but unlike other types of fats that your body can make, you can get these fats only if you eat them. The average western diet has more omega-6 than it should in relation to the amount of omega-3. You should make an effort to include more food containing omega-3 in your diet.

## How Do I Know Which Packaged Foods to Buy?

Most packaged foods have a label that gives the nutrition facts of the food. You may have noticed people in the grocery store studying the sides of boxes before they put them in their buggies. Have you ever wondered what it all means?

By reading the label, you can determine what is best for you to buy. See the boxes for examples.

The "% daily value" tells you the percentage of the total daily amount of this nutrient that is in one serving of this product. For example, the amount of fat in one serving of this bread is 3% of the total amount of fat you should eat during the day. For more information, go to www.healthyeatingisin store.ca (a Web site of the Canadian Diabetes Association and Dietitians of Canada). A Web site to help understand labels in the United States (which are slightly different) can be found at www.cfsan.fda.gov/~dms/foodlab.html.

---

**Reading Labels 1: A Multigrain bread**

| Nutrition Facts | |
|---|---|
| Per 2 slices | |
| **Amount** | **% Daily Value** |
| **Calories** 110 | |
| **Fat** 1.5 g | 3% |
| Saturated 0.3 g | 2% |
| + Trans 0 g | |
| **Cholesterol** 0 g | |
| **Sodium** 220 mg | 8% |
| **Carbohydrate** 20 g | 7% |
| Fiber 2 g | 8% |
| Sugars 1 g | |
| **Protein** 5 g | |
| | |
| Vitamin A 0%  Vitamin C 0% | |
| Calcium 0%  Iron 8% | |

According to the label, 2 slices of the loaf have 110 calories.

The fat content is 1.5 g and only 0.3 g of that is saturated fat. There are no trans fats.

One serving contains 20 g of carbohydrate in total, but you can subtract the fiber from it as that will just pass through you, and count one serving as 18 g of carbohydrates.

The other nutrients are important for people who have other health considerations and individual needs, such as a salt restriction.

**Reading Labels 2: A Cereal**

| Nutrition Facts | |
| --- | --- |
| Per 3/4 cup (30 g) | |
| **Amount** | **% Daily Value** |
| Calories 170 | |
| **Fat** 1 g | 2% |
| Saturated 0.2 g | 1% |
| + Trans 0 g | |
| **Cholesterol** 0 g | |
| **Sodium** 250 mg | 10% |
| Potassium 110 mg | 3% |
| **Carbohydrates** 39 g | 13% |
| Fiber 2 g | 9% |
| Sugars 10 g | |
| Starch 27 g | |
| **Protein** 4 g | |
| Vitamin A 0% Vitamin C 0% | |
| Calcium 0% Iron 0% | |

This product lists 3/4 of a cup as one serving with 170 calories.

There is only 1 g of fat and only 0.2 g of it is saturated fat.

There are 39 g of carbohydrate, but you can subtract the fiber as it passes through, so the total is 37 g.

You might want to look for a cereal that has a high fiber content.

This cereal is fairly high in carbohydrate. If you had 3/4 cup of it for breakfast, you have used 37 g of your total carb for the meal and more if you add milk. Look for cereals that have fewer carbohydrates per serving and preferably higher amounts of fiber that you can subtract from the total carbohydrate.

### Are Sweeteners Safe?

Sweeteners can be either nutritive or non-nutritive. Non-nutritive sweeteners are also known as "artificial sweeteners" and do not raise your blood glucose. There are several types of sweeteners and all are safe to use with the exception of two that should not be used when pregnant or breast-feeding: saccharin and cyclamate.

- aspartame (Nutrasweet, Equal);
- sucralose (Splenda);
- saccharin (Hermesetas);
- cyclamate (Sucaryl or Sugar Twin);
- acesulflame potassium (Sunett).

Health Canada has published the safe daily limits for the intake of these substances. This information is available on the Health Canada Web site. People who use a lot of artificial sweeteners should be aware of the recommended levels. Parents and caregivers should be particularly careful giving children these sweeteners because their smaller body size reduces the amount of the sweetener they should have.

The nutritive group of sweeteners is the sugar alcohol group: mannitol, maltitol, sorbitol, isomalt, and xylitol. These are not artificial sweeteners and can affect your blood glucose. These sugar alcohols are absorbed by your body but only about half as well as "real" sugar. Depending on the amount used, they can increase your blood glucose level. They are used in products such as chewing gum, sugar-free hard candies, sugar-reduced syrups, some jams, and chocolate. When you eat more than 10 grams of sugar alcohols in a day, you may experience abdominal cramps and diarrhea.

Claims on some food products may make you think a product has very little sugar. There are, however, only certain claims that food companies are allowed to make. To see what the claims mean see Appendix One.

At first, meal planning can sound overwhelming. Start with just one of the suggestions in this chapter and, after you have mastered that, move on to something else. Try to meet with a dietitian who will be able to clear up your questions and help you make healthy choices. Above all, remember that spreading out your meals and snacks through the day and eating moderate amounts are keys to healthy eating.

## Physical Activity

Exercise or physical activity is good for you! It builds strength in your muscles and bones, gives you better balance and a feeling of well being, reduces stress, helps you sleep better and, yes, even improves sex!

For people with type 2 diabetes, there are added benefits. Physical activity decreases your resistance to insulin so your insulin works better. An exercising muscle cell needs less insulin than an inactive muscle, so smaller amounts of insulin go further in someone who is physically active. If your own insulin works better, you may not need as much medication and your blood glucose levels can get closer to your target. In addition, regular physical activity has a good effect on the fats in your blood, improving the good cholesterol and often reducing the bad cholesterol. Increased physical activity lowers the risk that people with diabetes have for cardiac disease by improving blood glucose and blood fat (lipid) levels.

If you have type 1 diabetes, you are usually not resistant to insulin. The main benefit of exercise for you is to increase your sense of well-being and to decrease your risk of cardiac disease, such as a heart attack. You will need to discuss adjustments to your insulin dose and/or food intake to compensate for your physical activity. See Chapter Eight for an example of this.

### George's story

George does not like to exercise. He used to play hockey when he was young but now he thinks he is active enough at work and besides, when he gets home, he is too tired to go to the gym or even for a walk. Sometimes he finds he is short of breath after climbing the stairs, and says "I am out of shape" but in a moment he feels better and forgets about it. George always thought that he got enough exercise at work. He now realizes that he is really not that physically active and should do more to meet the recommendations for people with diabetes. He talks it over with his wife and they decide to walk together after supper every evening for 30 minutes. At first they find it difficult and have to encourage each other to keep at it. Soon, however, they look forward to this time together and the improved health they both experience as a result.

George is typical of many people as they get older. You may have been very active when younger, playing a sport, playing with the children, or just keeping in shape. Often, as you get busier and busier with family and career, the time spent on physical activity becomes shorter and shorter to make time for other important things. However, you are jeopardizing your health by cutting out the activity.

**How Much Do I Have to Do?**
Probably less than you think! The more active you are in your day-to-day life, the better. Housecleaning, walking to and from work, shopping, and chasing after small children all count as activity.

Most associations, like the Canadian Diabetes Association (CDA), recommend a minimum of 150 minutes a week of moderate to vigorous aerobic activity with no more than two consecutive days without activity. This could be about 30 minutes five days a week or 50 to 60 minutes three days a week and you don't even have to do it all at once. You could walk for 15 minutes before work and 15 minutes after work. Perhaps that means parking further away from your workplace or getting off the bus one stop earlier and walking the rest of the way. If you work in a building with an elevator, try walking up one or down two flights of stairs.

Aerobic activities are those where your muscles are active and you are working your cardiovascular system. Walking, biking, swimming, jogging, and dancing are all aerobic exercise. The other kind of activity that is good for you is resistance training. That means things like stretching, pushing against something like a wall, or weight lifting. It is recommended that everyone do some resistance-type activity at least three times a week for at least 10 minutes. Usually it means using different muscle groups in repetition eight times for three sets. The trainers at a local YMCA or exercise facility will be able to get you started. You may even be able to do it at home with an exercise tape.

**Before You Start to Exercise**

1. If you have not been physically active recently you should check with your doctor before you start. Your doctor should make sure that your heart is healthy and that your blood pressure is at a good level for you to increase your activity level. The doctor will also check that your feet are healthy and that you have good sensation in them. If you have lost some sensation in your feet, you might be at higher risk of developing a blister or sore without realizing it. The doctor will also examine your eyes or ask you to go for an eye exam since unrecognized changes in the retina might be present that could put vision at risk with sudden changes in activity and heart rate. These changes are rarely present unless glucose levels have been very poorly controlled or diabetes has been present a long time.

2. Wear comfortable, well-fitted shoes. Shoes should provide good support, with either tie-up or Velcro closings. They should be rounded at the front and have a high enough toe box to allow your toes to move. If you are not sure whether your shoes fit well, take your shoe off, stand up, and put your foot on a piece of paper. Trace your foot, then put the shoe

on the tracing and see if your foot goes outside your tracing. Do this for both feet, as often people have one foot larger than the other. If your shoe goes outside the tracing, it means your shoe is too tight and your foot is being squeezed.

3. Socks are also important. When you are active, your feet will likely sweat. You need socks that will draw the moisture away from your feet. If your feet are wet, the skin becomes soft and is more likely to break down. Also, be sure your socks fit and that the seam is not causing a ridge on your foot. You can buy socks that have no seams and no elastic in the top.

4. If you are on insulin or medications for your diabetes that may cause your glucose to fall too low, check your blood glucose. Any activity can cause your glucose level to drop so you want to know where it is before you start. You should also check when you finish exercising and a couple of hours later.

5. If you are on tablets, you may want to see how effective your after-dinner walk was in lowering you evening glucose compared to nights you don't walk. Take some fast-acting sugar source, such as glucose tablets, a juice box, or sugar cubes with you when exercising if your medications would put you at risk of a low blood glucose. If your blood glucose does drop too low, you need to be able to stop what you are doing and eat some fast-acting sugar right away. You may need to reduce your medications just before, during or after a regular exercise to avoid getting low blood glucose. Discuss with your doctor or diabetes educator whether you should adjust your medication for the type of exercise you will be doing.

If you are at risk of hypoglycemia, be sure that someone is either with you or knows when you are expected back.

There are some activities where it is safer to use a buddy system, such as wilderness hiking or swimming. Certain activities, where it is very difficult to stop and eat (for example, sky-diving or scuba diving), can be dangerous and should be undertaken with great caution.

---

## Check Blood Glucose around Exercising

Check before you start:

- If your blood glucose is too low, you will need to eat a fast-acting source of sugar to bring your glucose level up and then a snack to prevent low blood glucose during the activity.
- If your blood glucose level is higher than 14 mmol/L, you should likely put off the activity until your blood glucose is closer to your target range. If you have type 1 diabetes and your glucose is very high, intense activity might increase your stress hormones, which would result in your blood glucose levels going even higher.

Check during exercise.

Check immediately after exercise:

- If you need to eat something to replenish the glucose you have burned off during the exercise.

Check a few hours after:

- The blood glucose–lowering effect of exercise may not happen for a few hours, so you may be surprised by a low blood glucose several hours after the exercise or the following morning.

---

If you take medication to lower your blood glucose, you may need to reduce it on the days that you exercise, or within two hours before or after the exercise. Exercise helps the insulin that you have taken to act more effectively so that adjusting your insulin dose is very important in relation to exercise. Ask your doctor or diabetes educator how you should adjust your insulin and/or your meals on the days when you will be physically active.

**But I Don't Want to Exercise ...**

Starting something that you don't want to do is hard, but you don't have to do it alone. Most people find it is much easier to exercise if they do it with someone else. If a family member won't go with you, try joining a club. Ask a neighbor to join you. Get a dog—you won't be able to resist those big brown eyes asking for a walk! Most seniors' groups include people who walk or bike or swim. Many big malls support walking programs before the mall opens in the morning. Some even have a trail that has been measured and offer incentives. Call your local mall to see if such a program exists.

If you have arthritis in your knees or hips, exercising in water is beneficial. The water adds buoyancy and takes the weight off your joints. Even if you cannot swim, just walking back and forth in the shallow end is great exercise. Not only are you walking but also you have the resistance of the water pushing against you.

The other caution is not to bite off more than you can chew. Start slowly. If you have not been doing any physical activity, don't expect to be able to walk for 30 minutes without being exhausted and having all sorts of aches and pains. Take it

---

### Tips for Starting Your Exercise Activity

- Choose activities that you enjoy; there is a better chance you will continue.
- Start slowly, perhaps 10 minutes every day and increasing to 30 over 3 to 6 months.
- Try different activities to keep you from getting bored.
- Pick different activities to ensure all your muscle groups are being exercised.

The key is to develop the habit of being physically active, rather than inactive.

slowly; start with 5 minutes at a time and gradually work up—it won't take long and you will be proud of your progress!

### Should I get a pedometer?

A pedometer is a little meter that counts the number of steps you take, and can be worn on your belt. Pedometers are a great way to get motivated. Wear one for a few days and see how many steps you take on average. Then set yourself some goals. Perhaps set a goal to increase your total by 500 steps. Once you are comfortable at that level and reach it on most days, set another goal.

Some programs say you should take 10,000 steps a day. Unless you are already very active, you are probably far below that level. Don't let it worry you; any improvement you make and any increase in your daily activity will result in better health.

### But I am in a wheelchair ...

Being in a wheelchair or otherwise challenged does not mean you cannot be physically active. Look for ways you can get those muscles moving. Move your arms and shoulders around. Ask someone else to bend your legs back and forth, which will provide exercise for both of you.

Starting a program of physical activity is not easy and most people can think of many reasons they can put it off for another day. Being physically active does make a difference to your diabetes management, so think positively and start with something, even if only a few minutes a day. Soon you will see and feel the difference.

## Monitoring Your Blood Glucose

Checking your blood glucose at home is the one way you can know for sure how well you are managing your diabetes. You may think that you are doing the checks simply to please the doctor or diabetes educator, but really you should be doing them for yourself. You are the person in charge of your diabetes and you need to know what to do and how well you are doing. You have probably discussed a target range for your blood glucose with your doctor or diabetes educator. Be sure you know the targets for both before and after meals. How will you know if you are achieving those targets if you do not check yourself?

### Where Should Blood Glucose Levels Be?

Target ranges for blood glucose vary somewhat from country to country and should be determined individually. But, as a general rule, the following are safe levels for most people.

In Canada, it is recommended that blood glucose levels be low enough to achieve an A1C level of less than 7 percent. Target levels are currently set at the following levels:

- fasting and before a meal: 4–7 mmol/L (72–126 mg/dl);
- 2 hours after eating: 5–10 mmol/L (100–180 mg/dl).

If the A1C remains more than than 7 percent, after-meal targets may be lowered to 5–8 mmol/L (90–144 mg/dl). In young children, the elderly or those with significant heart disease, targets may have to be raised to avoid hypoglycemia. In pregnant women and those planning pregnancy, these targets should be lowered.

You should discuss with your doctor or diabetes team the specific target levels that are best for you.

*Jim's story*

> Jim was given a blood glucose meter some time ago but has
> fallen out of the habit of using it. He used it at first, but was
> not sure what the numbers meant or if he should do anything
> about them so it all seemed to be a waste of time. And, besides,
> he didn't like pricking his finger. The last time he went to the
> doctor, the doctor asked him about his glucose levels at home.
> Jim is now wondering if he should start checking again and, if
> so, why and when.

**When Should You Check?**

When you check will depend on many things:

- what you want to know;
- what medication you are on;
- what changes are happening in your life;
- whether or not you are sick.

Checking should be used to give you specific information about
what is happening to the glucose you take in and the treatment you are on.

The Canadian Diabetes Association (CDA) and the American Diabetes Association (ADA) have published some basic
guidelines about the amount of testing a person should do.
CDA and ADA agree that people with type 1 diabetes or type
2 diabetes taking more than 1 injection of insulin a day should
check at least three times a day. The CDA states that most
people with type 2 diabetes who are on once-daily insulin or
oral medication should check at least once a day. More frequent checking is recommended when information is required
to make behavioral or treatment adjustments. The ADA makes

no specific recommendation for the number of times a person with type 2 diabetes should check but suggests that checking should be done to adjust behavior or treatment as well. Everyone who has diabetes can learn something by checking at specific times of the day. The more you know about how your body manages your glucose, the better you will be able to keep your blood glucose levels within your target range.

*Type 2—healthy eating and activity only*
If you manage your diabetes with healthy eating and activity only, that is without tablets or insulin, you might be able to get a picture of your blood glucose range by checking before breakfast and one to two hours after your largest meal of the day, and by doing this two or three days a month. If those results are all within your target range, you can be somewhat assured that you are managing well. You might also want to know how certain foods affect your blood glucose. For instance, you have a favorite dessert you want to have on occasion, but you are worried it might push your glucose level too high. Try checking your blood glucose before you eat it and again one to two hours after you eat it, to see what difference the dessert made. Your blood glucose should increase by about 2–3 mmol/L (35–55 mg/dl) after a meal. If you find your level was too high after the favorite dessert, try having a smaller piece next time, or perhaps going for a walk before eating it so you start the meal with a lower blood glucose.

*Type 2—oral medications and/or insulin*
If you take oral medications and/or insulin for diabetes you will want to use your meter checks to determine how well your medication is working. In order to do this, find the peak action

time of your medication. Some oral medications and some insulins work within one to two hours after they are taken; others take longer to work. To be sure that your glucose level is within your target, it is important to check your blood glucose at the time the medication should be working maximally. If the result is too high, then consider what you ate for the last meal. The dose will have been set according to your eating habits or the expected amount of food. If you have eaten a large meal or one with more starch or sweets than usual, the result might be a higher blood glucose level. If you have eaten less carbohydrate than your meal plan suggests, the blood glucose level might be lower. Before deciding that your oral medication or insulin is not working well enough or working too well, ask yourself if you are making the right choices regarding the type and amount of food.

*Type 1—insulin*
If you have type 1 diabetes, you are probably learning how to or are already adjusting your mealtime insulin according to your blood glucose level and the size of the meal you are going to eat. If you are doing this, then you should be checking before each meal and at various times after a meal to see if you made the correct adjustment to the dose.

*Advantages of checking your own blood glucose*
- You will know the effect of food eaten, by checking before the meal and one to two hours after the meal.
- You will know the effect of physical activity by checking before, during, and at various intervals several hours following the activity.
- You can determine whether how you are feeling is due to your blood glucose level.
- You can check for and recognize a hypoglycemic event,

in order to be able to treat it early. (Chapter Eight has a description of this and other consequences of high and low blood sugar levels.)

- You can check for and recognize when the blood glucose levels are rising and be able to avoid the more serious consequences of diabetic ketoacidosis (DKA) or hyperglycemic hyperosmolar nonketotic state (HHS). (See Chapter Eight.)

The results from your glucose meter help you, your doctor and your diabetes educator decide about management recommendations, changes in medication, or your meal timing or portions. Working together, you can learn about the effects of meals and activities on your blood glucose levels.

**Interpreting Your Results**

Changes to medication should never be based on just one or two results. You need to check frequently enough to show a pattern. Some people check four or more times a day. But, if this is too much for you, there are other ways to show a pattern over a short time period. You should try to get two or three results for each time in a week. This means that one day you could check before breakfast and before supper, the next day before lunch and before going to bed. The next day you might do a couple of checks two hours after meals. After about ten days of rotating your checking, you will be able to see a pattern in your results. Of course, if you check more frequently you will see a pattern sooner.

When looking at your logbook or diary, the first thing is to get an overview. Are the results all above your target range? Are they below your target? Do they jump around like a roller coaster? Remember that your levels will not be exactly the same all the time; there will always be some ups and downs, but they should stay within your target range overall.

Once you have an overview of your pattern, look for results that are below target. It is ***important to solve the problem of low blood glucose first.***

- Are you having lows at the same time of day?
- Are they always after you exercise?
- Do you see a pattern to them?
- Do you know why you had the low?

For instance, you might have skipped a meal. If you know the reason for the lows, you know how to prevent them from happening again. Write the reasons in your logbook to help you remember. If you do not know the reason, you should talk to your doctor or diabetes educator. You might need a change in your medication. If you do not have any low results, look for results above the target range.

- What time of day are they?
- Can you think of a reason for them?

Again, write down the reason while it is fresh in your mind.

Blood glucose checking allows you to know what your blood glucose level is at any time. This can be very useful to assist in making decisions about your daily activities. However, you need to learn how to interpret your results and how to make changes to either food intake or medication to improve your levels. Diabetes educators or physicians are the usual people to do this type of teaching.

**Recording Results**
Although most meters have memories and the contents of these can be downloaded onto a computer, it is very helpful if you

keep a handwritten logbook indicating your medications doses, too. Sometimes the doctor or diabetes educator will mark in the logbook the times to record a result. When logbooks are well kept, legible, and accurate, it is much easier to make decisions based on the results.

Comments added to specific results are also very useful. For instance, if dinner was later than usual or a low result was the result of activity, it should be recorded at the side. This will help you, the doctor, or educator decide if there should be changes made.

*Jim's story*
After discussion with his health care provider, Jim has decided to check before and after several meals for the next week. Here are his results. What do you notice about them?

| | Before Breakfast | After Breakfast | Before Lunch | After Lunch | Before Supper | After Supper |
|---|---|---|---|---|---|---|
| Mon | 10.2 mmol/L (183 mg/dl) | 14.8 (266) | | | 8.6 (154) | 12.5 (225) |
| Tues | | | 10.6 (190) | 11.4 (205) | | |
| Wed | 11.3 mmol/L (203 mg/dl) | 15.1 (272) | | | 7.9 (142) | 10.3 (185) |
| Thurs | | | 9.8 (176) | 12.5 (225) | | |

Note: Values for blood glucose results are given two ways. In Canada, meters read in mmol/L; in the United States, meters read in mg/dl. To convert from one to the other, multiply mmol/L by 18 to get mg/dl or divide mg/dl by 18 to get mmol/L.

• They are fairly consistent—ranging from 7.9 to 15.1 mmol/L (142–272 mg/dl) but most are a little over 10 mmol/L (180 mg/dl).
• There are no results lower than 4 mmol/L (72 mg/dl).

- The before-meal results are consistently higher than 7 mmol/L (120 mg/dl).

With such levels, what should Jim do?
   First, Jim should try to figure out why his results are always high before meals.

- Is he taking his medication as prescribed?
- Is he eating more carbs than he should?
- Is he less active than last month when his results were lower?
- Has he been sick or under unusual stress?

If a reason for the elevated results cannot be found, then, in all likelihood, a different dosage or medication is needed. When this type of situation occurs, it would be best for Jim to take his records to his doctor and ask for advice. He should not wait it out hoping that they will get better on their own.

**Tips for Accurate Checking**
Blood glucose meters give very accurate results when they are used properly. Here are some of the factors that relate to the meter and/or test strip equipment.

*Getting the drop of blood*
- Your hands should be clean. If there is a sugary substance on your fingers, such as juice, candy, etc., your reading may be inaccurately high.
- Squeezing your finger for blood must be done gently, starting at the base of the finger and gently pushing the blood out to the tip of the finger. When your finger is squeezed too firmly at the tip, the sample will contain fluid other than just blood, which will result in an inaccurate reading.
- An adequate drop of blood must be obtained for accu-

rate checking. Some meters detect when the strip has not received enough blood to give an accurate reading (underfill detection). Meters with this feature will give an error message or will not register the result. If the meter does not have this feature it might still display a reading, which could be inaccurate.

### Coding the meter

Coding the meter means setting the meter to match a batch of strips. Some meters do this automatically, some require the user to manually code them. Blood glucose meters that require coding by the user warn that inaccurate results may result if the meter is not correctly coded. Review each manufacturer's product manual to ensure you know how to code your meter correctly. Some meters do not require coding.

### Storage of strips and strip stability

- Strips must not be left open to the air.
- Strips that are foil-wrapped are good until the expiry date indicated on the package, provided that they are opened only at the time of use. Strips in a container must be left in the container with the top closed.
- Containers have an expiry date on them, and unopened strips are good until the expiry date. However, once the container is opened the strips are good only for three or six months, depending on the brand.
- Mark on the container when it was opened.

### Temperature

- Meters and test strips that are too hot or too cold will not work. If your meter is too cold, allow it time to warm up before trying to use it. For most meters, the optimal temperature range is 10–40°C (50–104°F).

## Alternate-Site Testing

- Alternate-site testing, that is poking an area other than the fingertips for a drop of blood, is recommended only when your blood glucose is not moving up or down too much.
- The sites usually used are the forearm and the hand where it is thicker at the base of the thumb or small finger. The advantage of these sites is that they have fewer nerve endings, so there may be less discomfort when testing. The disadvantage is that there is a delay in glucose getting into the blood in the subcutaneous tissue. *When glucose is on the way up or down, the glucose value measured at these sites will lag behind the levels in the fingertips.*
- Thus, fingertip testing is preferred after meals, when medication is peaking, or anytime hypoglycemia is suspected. Not all meters are approved for alternate site testing; you should consult the user manuals for details.

## Continuous Glucose Monitoring Devices

- There are more and more devices coming to market that are able to measure "interstitial" fluid glucose levels. These devices require the person insert a small catheter into tissue under the skin of the abdomen. The newer sensors have integrated radio signaling that sends information about the glucose result either to an insulin pump or to a receiver that looks like a cell phone, on a 24-hour basis.
- There is a need to let the sensor "calibrate" or establish itself under the skin. This may take from 2 to 12 hours and requires a finger-prick check to tell the sensor your glucose level. This means you need to do a fingertip check about two to four times a day to re-calibrate.
- Throughout the day for as long as the sensor lasts (about 3 to 5 days), it is possible to look at the readout and know where your glucose level is, as well as whether it is on the

way up or down and how quickly it is moving up or down. The lag seen in alternate-site testing is also evident with this method. Thus, in any situation where glucose may be falling or rising, it is necessary to do a fingertip check as well, since capillary glucose is closer to what the blood glucose really is and changes of diet or insulin may be needed.

• At present, it is mainly used to problem solve rather than for routine care. Clearly, since the sensors are expensive and do not last long, this is not a solution for everyone. It is, however, the next step toward closing the loop between sensing the glucose and the automatic delivery of the correct amount of insulin as the islets in our pancreas do when diabetes is not present.

## How to Be Sure Your Meter Is Accurate

To ensure the accuracy of your meter, you should take it with you when you go to the lab for a blood test. After the blood is drawn from your arm, do a fingertip poke and usual blood check. Write the result in your logbook and circle it so you will remember which check it was. Then when you get the result from the lab test, compare it to your circled result. When you are fasting, there is more likely to be a better match between your lab result and your meter result. Generally, there should be no more than a 20 percent difference between your meter and the lab results. That means if your meter result was 7.5 mmol/L, the lab result should have been between 6 and 9 mmol/L.

Example:  $7.5 \times .2 = 1.5$
$7.5 - 1.5 = 6$
$7.5 + 1.5 = 9$

If your meter is not giving results in a 20 percent range, contact the manufacturer.

## Things to Look for in a Meter

| Consideration | Reasoning |
|---|---|
| Does the meter have to be coded? | Coding is done by either putting a chip in the meter or scrolling through numbers on the screen to get a match to the new container of strips. It takes a few seconds and must be done every time a new container of strips is opened. Some meters automatically code themselves when a strip is inserted. |
| How much blood do you need? | Unfortunately all meters do require a drop of blood, but the amount is different from one to another. For some the drop size is about the size of a pinhead. |
| How fast will you get a result? | Some meters will give a result in as little as five seconds. |
| Can you poke somewhere other than your fingertips? | Usually the meters that work with the smallest drop of blood are the ones approved for alternate-site testing. It is often a little more difficult to get blood from your arm or elsewhere. |
| How big is the memory? And does it have special features? | Some meters not only remember the last results you got, but also put them into graphs or sort them according to time of day, whether it is before or after a meal, etc. If you are looking for patterns and making changes to your diabetes management plan, then you might want a meter that will help you see this sort of information easily. |
| Will it connect to my computer? | Almost all meters will connect and download information to specific programs on the computer. The programs are available from the manufacturers. Downloads can be helpful if you want to print off a list of results to take to your doctor, and they will give you useful graphs that can help you to understand why or where your blood glucose levels are in or out of target range. |
| Do I have to put in a strip each time I use the meter? | There are some meters that provide the strips in a canister or disk that fits right into the meter. The canister or disk holds a number of strips so you do not have to insert a strip each time. With these meters, as soon as you turn the meter on, a strip pokes out. |
| How are the strips packaged or how big is the container? | Containers are usually quite small, with lids that either flip open or screw open. Some strips are packaged individually in foil. |
| Do all strips cost the same? | This will vary from country to country but they are all more or less the same. Some private insurance policies do cover strips. Some provinces in Canada have programs to help with the cost of strips. |
| What is the cost of the meter? | The cost of meters varies depending on where you are and if there are special promotions under way. Some private insurance policies may cover the cost of the meter. |

**Which Meter Should I Buy?**

There are several things to consider when looking for a meter and, while it is fair to say that all meters will give accurate results when used properly, certain models have advantages over others for some people.

If you are not sure which meter is best for you and/or you have special needs or difficulties, discuss with your diabetes educator or pharmacist which meter would be best for you. Monitoring is a powerful tool but, as with any tool, it works only if you know how to use it.

## Checking for Ketones

When your body does not have enough glucose for energy it starts to break down fat. In doing so ketones are produced (see Chapter Eight). Ketones are converted to acids in the liver if not enough insulin is present. They then enter into the blood stream and change the chemical balance in the blood. Your body tries to get rid of the ketones/ketoacids by passing them out in your urine. You might have ketones in your urine if you did not eat all day or you did some very strenuous exercise. If you have enough insulin, the ketones will be cleared by your liver and into your urine, causing no problem.

If you are ill and the amount of insulin that you have available is very low, the ketones cannot be cleared well. If the amount of ketones in your urine is moderate to large and if your blood glucose is also higher than normal, you may be developing ketoacidosis. See Chapter Eight.

You can check your urine for ketones by dipping a special strip in the urine and checking the color. You can also check your blood for ketones using a special meter and a finger prick similar to blood glucose checking. Checking for ketones in your blood is more accurate than urine ketone testing and will show rising levels earlier than they would be seen in the urine.

You should test for ketones:

- during illness;
- if your blood glucose is more than 14 mmol/L (252 mg/dl);
- if you are using a pump and suspect a problem with insulin delivery;
- in the presence of symptoms of ketoacidosis such as fruity-smelling breath, abdominal pain, or feeling very ill (see Chapter Eight).

If you have moderate or more ketones in the urine, get medical help quickly.

Women with gestational diabetes are sometimes asked to test their urine for ketones. In pregnancy, ketones will form more quickly than in the non-pregnant state if the time between meals is too long. Checking ketones helps tell your health care team if your meal plan is adequate; it is important that pregnant women have adequate nutrition at the right time to ensure ideal development of the baby. These women are not at risk of ketoacidosis.

## Checking Your Urine for Glucose

You usually have no glucose in your urine. When your blood glucose level is higher than about 10 mmol/L (180 mg/dl), the kidneys will not be able to keep the glucose in. The level at which you spill glucose into your urine is called the *renal threshold*.

You will see glucose in your urine check only if your blood glucose level is over your renal threshold. The benefits of urine checking are limited because:

- You do not know what your renal threshold is.
- Your renal threshold may vary for instance during pregnancy and as you age.
- A negative result just tells you that you are below your renal threshold but not if you are in the target range for blood glucose.
- You cannot determine if your blood glucose is too low; a urine check result that is negative for glucose indicates only that your blood glucose is below your renal threshold.
- Your urine glucose may reflect what your blood glucose was about two hours before—it takes time for the blood to circulate through your kidneys and the glucose to spill into your urine.
- Some medications and vitamins can alter the color of the urine and cause false results.

Checking your urine for glucose is better than not checking your glucose at all. If you have positive urine checks, it means that your blood glucose is above your *renal threshold* and therefore above the target level. If your urine is positive for glucose on an ongoing basis, talk to your doctor or a member of your health care team as you may need a change in medication.

# Medications Other Than Insulin

*The information in this chapter is a basic overview of available medication. You must always discuss starting or changing any medication with your doctor.*

Medications play an important role in the management of type 2 diabetes. As you have learned from earlier chapters, in type 2 diabetes there are two things going on. First, you are resistant to the effects of insulin in your body and, second, you are making less insulin than your body needs. When first diagnosed, you may be able to manage diabetes by revising your eating habits and becoming more physically active. Your new eating habits will result in less glucose being taken in at any one time, and the exercise will improve the sensitivity of your cells to the insulin, keeping your blood glucose levels within targets.

Eventually, however, the blood glucose will not stay within target levels as the amount of insulin produced continues to fall. At this point there are a number of oral medications that can be tried to enhance the effects of your healthy meal plan and improved physical activity.

The first oral medications for treating diabetes were developed in the 1940s. None of these medications are insulin and they do not act in the same way as insulin. Oral medications are not a form of oral insulin.

When considering how the oral medications work in your body, it helps to understand how your body controls the glucose. Although some of this has been explained in Chapter One, the figures on pages 92, 93, and 95 will help you understand the interactions between the organs responsible for keeping your glucose normal, what goes wrong with diabetes and how, and where each of the medications used for diabetes seems to work. Each medication acts primarily at one site or by using one mechanism, so they will be described by their mode of action.

### Organs and Tissues Involved in Keeping Glucose Levels Steady

The diagram on page 92 shows all the organs that help to keep the glucose levels normal in your body.

- stomach and intestine—where the digestive process occurs; some glucose is absorbed into the blood from the stomach, the rest from the intestine. The stomach and intestine also release hormones called incretins that help to make insulin work in response to a meal and help tell our brain centers that we have eaten.
- pancreas—releases insulin in response to levels of glucose in the blood.

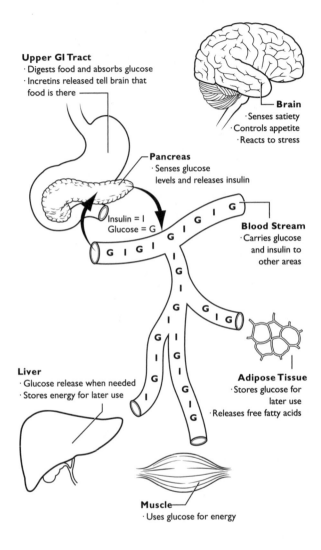

**Upper GI Tract**
· Digests food and absorbs glucose
· Incretins released tell brain that
  food is there

**Brain**
· Senses satiety
· Controls appetite
· Reacts to stress

**Pancreas**
· Senses glucose
  levels and releases insulin

Insulin = I
Glucose = G

**Blood Stream**
· Carries glucose
  and insulin to
  other areas

**Liver**
· Glucose release when needed
· Stores energy for later use

**Adipose Tissue**
· Stores glucose for
  later use
· Releases free fatty acids

**Muscle**
· Uses glucose for energy

- liver—stores glucose and releases it when blood levels drop too low.
- muscles—use glucose from the blood to make energy.
- adipose (fat) tissue—stores glucose and releases it when

levels are low; it also releases substances that tell our brain that we have eaten.

- brain—tells you if you are hungry or not, which affects the amount and kind of food you eat.

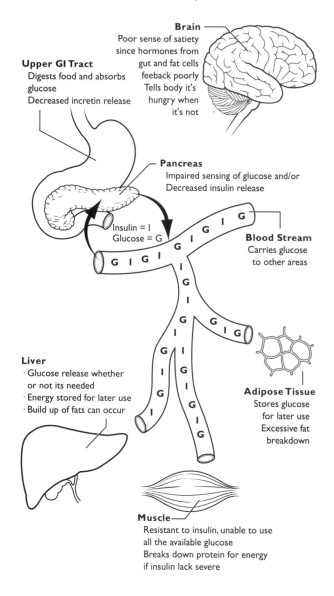

**Brain**
Poor sense of satiety
since hormones from
gut and fat cells
feeback poorly
Tells body it's
hungry when
it's not

**Upper GI Tract**
Digests food and absorbs
glucose
Decreased incretin release

**Pancreas**
Impaired sensing of glucose and/or
Decreased insulin release

Insulin = I
Glucose = G

**Blood Stream**
Carries glucose
to other areas

**Liver**
· Glucose release whether
  or not its needed
· Energy stored for later use
· Build up of fats can occur

**Adipose Tissue**
Stores glucose
for later use
Excessive fat
breakdown

**Muscle**
Resistant to insulin, unable to use
all the available glucose
Breaks down protein for energy
if insulin lack severe

## Some Processes That Go Wrong in Type 2 Diabetes

- pancreas—beta cells may not release enough insulin;
- liver—may release too much glucose.
- muscles—may be resistant to insulin so that glucose cannot enter;
- adipose (fat) tissue—may release too much glucose and send fatty acids to the liver, which pushes extra glucose release even when not needed.
- brain—may receive and thus send incorrect signals regarding the need for food.

## Mechanisms of Action of Medications Used to Treat Type 2 Diabetes

The medications other than insulin can be grouped into the following five categories by their action:

- slows gut absorption of glucose and/or fats from the gut;
- stimulates the release of insulin from the beta cell;
- reduces the amount of glucose the liver produces, helping to reduce the degree of insulin resistance.;
- reduces insulin resistance in muscle and fat cells increasing the action of insulin;
- improves the responsiveness of the pancreas to the blood glucose level.

Which medication will be started first and whether or not more than one will be started depends on your needs. If your blood glucose levels are very high you might be asked to start with two different medications at the same time. For instance, you might take one that makes you more sensitive to your insulin and another that stimulates your pancreas to give you

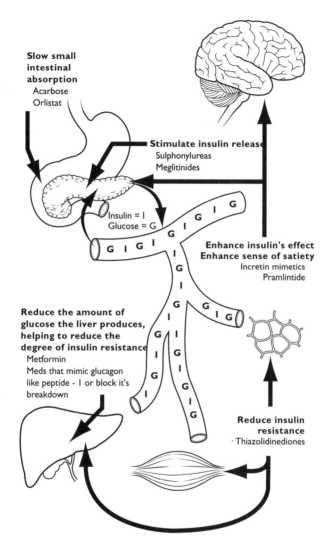

Slow small
intestinal
absorption
Acarbose
Orlistat

Stimulate insulin release
Sulphonylureas
Meglitinides

Insulin = I
Glucose = G

Enhance insulin's effect
Enhance sense of satiety
Incretin mimetics
Pramlintide

Reduce the amount of
glucose the liver produces,
helping to reduce the
degree of insulin resistance
Metformin
Meds that mimic glucagon
like peptide - I or block it's
breakdown

Reduce insulin
resistance
· Thiazolidinediones

more insulin. Together this would give you more available insulin and the insulin would work better.

Some people even take one from each of three or four categories. Two medications from the same category are not usually taken together as there would be no added advantage from the second. If blood glucose is not at target levels after you have tried two or three oral medications, it is time to switch to insulin. Sometimes insulin can be used early to correct very high glucose levels and then oral agents will be more effective, even if the insulin is stopped.

### What Does Generics Mean?

- *generic name*—the chemical name of the compound;
- *brand name*—the name given by the company.

All medications have both a generic name and a brand name. There may be many brand names for the same generic name depending on how many companies make it. In this chapter, only the generic names have been used, although some brand names have been listed in the Table of Drug Names on page 250. If you are not sure what you are taking, ask your doctor or pharmacist.

"Generics" is a common term that refers to medications made by many companies and sold at lower cost once the patent of the brand name medication has run out.

The following information represents a brief overview of the various oral medications used in the treatment of diabetes. Speak with your doctor, pharmacist, or diabetes educator to obtain more precise information about the medications that you take.

## Medications That Slow the Absorption of Glucose or Fat from the Gut

### Alpha Glucosidase Inhibitor

- This medication when taken right before a meal slows the absorption of certain complex sugars in the bowel. This means that the glucose rise after a meal will not be as fast, since these sugars will be absorbed slowly throughout the intestine. This medication can cause abdominal gas and bloating.

The expected decrease in A1C from this medication when used alone is 0.5–0.8 percent.

| Generic Name | Dose | Contraindications | When to Take It | Comments |
|---|---|---|---|---|
| acarbose | Usually started with 25–50 mg at one meal and gradually built up. Maximum dose: 300 mg/day (100 mg before each meal). | Severe kidney or liver damage, chronic intestinal disorder, pregnancy and nursing mothers. | Must be taken with the first bite of the meal. | Abdominal gas may be minimized by starting with a low dose and very gradually increasing the dose. |

This medication will not cause hypoglycemia by itself. However, if you take it with other medication that can cause hypoglycemia, only certain forms of sugar can be used to treat the hypoglycemia. This medication blocks absorption of "classic" sugar-bowl sugar. Therefore, if your blood glucose is low, you need to take actual glucose (as in glucose tablets from the pharmacy) or the sugar in milk (lactose) to bring your glucose back up.

### Orlistat

When taken right before a meal this medication slows the absorption of the fat components in the food. This helps reduce the speed of the increase in glucose after a meal. When too much fat is present in the meal, the medication has considerable side effects, thus encouraging you to eat less fatty meals.

This medication can:

- cause abdominal gas and bloating;
- cause loose bowel movements or diarrhea;
- occasionally will cause incontinence of stool (involuntary loss of stool) if there is too much fat in the meal.

The expected decrease in A1C from this medication when used alone is 0.5–0.8 percent

| Generic Name | Dose | Contraindications | When to Take It | Comments |
|---|---|---|---|---|
| orlistat | Usually started with 50–100 mg at one meal and gradually built up. Maximum dose: 300 mg/day (100 mg before each meal). | Pregnancy and nursing mothers. | Taken during or up to one hour after a meal. | Digestive side effects may be minimized by reducing the fat in the food to very low amounts. |

## Medications That Stimulate the Release of Insulin from Beta Cells

There are two groups of these medications: the sulphonylureas and the meglitinides. In order for these medications to work, your beta cells have to be able to make insulin. These medications are not to be used in people with type 1 diabetes. Within each group there are several different medications with slightly different actions.

### Sulphonylureas

This group of medications stimulates your pancreas to release more insulin regardless of the level of glucose in your blood.

All sulphonylureas can cause:

- hypoglycemia (low blood glucose)
- weight gain—usually 1–4 kg initially, which then stabilizes
- sensitivity reactions—mild rash or rarely photosensitivity

Chlorpropamide can cause facial flushing with alcohol consumption. Rarely, some of these medications (primarily chlorpropamide) can lead to low sodium in the blood.

When used alone, this group of medications is likely to reduce the A1C by about 1.5 percent, but this may depend on how much beta-cell function remains, as the main function of this group is to stimulate insulin release.

| Generic Name | Dose | Contraindi-cations | When to Take It | Comments |
|---|---|---|---|---|
| tolbutamide | Usually started with 250–500 mg /day and increased to twice a day if blood glucose levels are not at target. Maximum dose: 2000 mg/day (usually 500 mg with meals). | Pregnancy, nursing mothers, kidney disease. | Take close to a meal or with food. | This medication is not used as frequently today as others. It is occasionally used in older people due to its shorter duration of action. |
| chlorpro-pamide | Usually started with 100 mg/day. Maximum dose: 500 mg/day. | Pregnancy, nursing mothers, kidney disease, elderly. | Take in the morning before breakfast. | Lasts a long time in the body so can build up and cause severe hypo-glycemia. Not used often. |
| glyburide | Usually started with 2.5–5 mg at breakfast. Maximum dose: 20 mg/day, usually as 10 mg at breakfast and supper. | Liver or kidney disease. (Pregnancy and nursing mothers) * | Take before meals. | Can last a long time in some people, which can result in severe hypoglycemia. |
| gliclazide | Usually started with 40–80 mg once daily. Maximum dose 320 mg/day usually divided between breakfast and supper. | Pregnancy, nursing mothers. | Take before meals. | Cleared more quickly than glyburide—can cause less hypo-glycemia. |
| gliclazide MR | Usually started with 30 mg once daily at breakfast. Maximum dose: 120 mg once a day. | Pregnancy, nursing mothers. | Take before breakfast. | As above with convenience of once-a-day dosing. |
| glimepiride | Usually started with 1–2 mg daily at breakfast. Maximum dose: 8 mg/day at breakfast. | Pregnancy, nursing mothers, kidney disease. | Take before breakfast. | |

*In some areas of the world this medication is used through some or all of the pregnancy although the long-term effects are not known.

## Meglitinides

Meglitinides also stimulate the pancreas to release more insulin, but work much faster and for a shorter time than the sulphonylureas. They should be taken immediately prior to a meal to target the rise in blood glucose following the meal.

Meglitinides can cause:

- hypoglycemia;
- weight gain, usually 1–3 kg initially, then stabilizes;
- rash (mild and rare).

If used alone, repaglinide is expected to reduce A1C by 1.5 percent, nateglinide by only 0.5 percent. Again this would depend on the remaining function of the beta cells.

| Generic Name | Dose | Contraindi-cations | When to Take It | Comments |
|---|---|---|---|---|
| nateglinide | Usually started at 120 mg with each meal. Maximum dose: 540 mg/day (180 mg at each meal). | Pregnancy, nursing mothers, children, liver disease. | 1–30 minutes before meal, skip dose if meal is skipped. | Duration of action (about 4 hours). |
| repaglinide | Usually started with 0.5 mg with each meal. Maximum dose: 4 mg per meal up to 4 meals a day. | Same as nateglinide. | Take 1–30 minutes before meal, skip dose if meal is skipped. | Duration of action (4–5 hours). |

# Medications That Help Reduce the Degree of Insulin Resistance

### Biguanide (Metformin)

This medication lowers fasting glucose levels by reducing the production and release of glucose from the liver. As mentioned previously, the liver stores excess glucose in several forms. When blood glucose levels are low or when stimulated by other hormones, the liver will release glucose as needed into the blood, which can be helpful. However, if insulin levels are low, the liver will release too much glucose. Metformin helps to restore lower and more-normal liver glucose release. It may also help the muscle cells to be less resistant to insulin, so the insulin you have will work better.

Biguanides can cause:

- abdominal cramping or diarrhea—usually this is minimized by starting with a low dose and gradually increasing as needed;
- risk of lactic acidosis that is very rare and seen only in those with severe kidney, liver, or heart disease;
- reduced absorption of vitamin $B_{12}$.

When used alone, metformin may be expected to reduce the A1C by about 1–2 percent.

| Generic Name | Dose | Contraindications | When to Take It | Comments |
|---|---|---|---|---|
| metformin | Usual started at 250 mg once or twice a day. Maximum dose: 2500 mg/day (usually as 1000 mg at breakfast and supper and 500 mg at lunch). | Kidney or liver disease, alcohol abuse, congestive heart failure or recent heart attack, respiratory failure *(Pregnancy and nursing mothers) | Take with meals. | May cause abdominal discomfort when first started, which usually stops in a short time if dose is started at low level and gradually increased. |

*In some areas of the world this medication is used through some or all of the pregnancy although the long-term effects are not known.

## Thiazolidinediones

These medications increase the action of insulin in the tissues by improving the sensitivity of the tissues to insulin. They do not give you more insulin but allow the insulin that you have to work better. Although they often have an effect that can be seen reasonably quickly, their full effect is not obvious for up to 12 weeks. Their effect on controlling glucose does not appear to decrease with time, as is often seen with sulphonylurea medications.

Thiazolidinediones can cause:

- fluid retention;
- weight gain up to 2 to 4 kg over 1–2 years;
- increased risk of congestive heart failure;
- increased risk of fractures; and
- possible increased risk of heart attacks for rosiglitazone.

Use of these medications can worsen either recognized or unrecognized heart failure. This would lead to swelling of the feet and ankles or edema and/or some shortness of breath with effort. If these symptoms occur, you should discontinue the medications and contact your doctor.

A recent academic review questioned the possibility that even without known heart disease, people taking rosiglitazone may be at higher risk of a myocardial infarction (heart attack) or other cardiovascular event. The same possible risk for heart attacks does not seem to be seen using pioglitzone. There may also be an increased risk of fractures, particularly in women on these drugs.

When used alone, thiazolidinediones can be expected to reduce A1C by 0.5–1.4 percent.

| Generic Name | Dose | Contraindi-cations | When to Take It | Comments |
|---|---|---|---|---|
| pioglitazone | Usually started at 15 mg/day. Maximum dose: 45 mg once daily. | Kidney or liver disease, heart failure, pregnancy. | Take at the same time each day with or without food. | May see some effect after 2 weeks but best effect not usually seen until 8–12 weeks after starting. |
| rosiglitazone | Usually started at 4 mg/day. Maximum dose: 8 mg/day usually split 4 mg at breakfast and 4 mg at supper. | Kidney or liver disease, heart failure, pregnancy. | Take at the same time each day with or without food. | May see some effect after 2 weeks but best effect not usually seen until 8–12 weeks after starting. **An increased risk of cardiovascular problems in some people on this medication.** |

# Medications That Enhance the Incretin System

As discussed in Chapter One, as part of the normal digestive process, hormones called incretins (gut hormones) are released and affect how you respond to the glucose in the food, as well as help feedback to the brain that you have eaten. This system has been called the incretin system.

**What's the Gut "Breaking System" or Incretin System?**
When you eat, the body sends signals from sensors in the gut (stomach, intestines, pancreas) to help you deal with the food. The system could be described as the gut "breaking system." This system has many actions, including:

- slowing the passage of food through the gastrointestinal tract to allow it to be better absorbed;
- telling you that you have eaten enough by sending a message to the satiety center in your brain;
- being sure the amount of insulin released is right for the amount of food you just ate; and
- helping the body decide how much glucose from the food goes to the muscle cells and how much gets stored in the liver; and
- lowering the effect of glucagon (the hormone that tells the liver to release stored glucose if you need it).

In addition there are indications that incretins may have additional effects such as:

- improving the first-phase insulin release that is usually lost early in type 2 diabetes;

- helping the body to maintain the beta cells, or cells that make insulin, ensuring that they live as long as possible;
- helping the body regenerate new beta cells if it needs them.

The hormone that is the most important of those naturally occurring in the system is called glucagon-like protein-1 or GLP-1. GLP-1 can markedly improve the glucose levels at the same time encourage stable weight or weight loss. However it needs to be given continuously by IV, and is broken down very quickly by an enzyme (DPP-IV) in the body. The following developments appear to solve these limitations.

## Incretin Mimetics

*GLP-1 agonists (molecules that work like GLP-1)*
The Gila monster (one of only two species of highly venomous lizards) has a hormone in its saliva that is very similar to GLP-1, but which is not broken down by the enzyme DPP-IV. A product called exenatide has been synthesized to mimic this hormone. As of 2007, although available in many countries including the United States and Europe, it is not yet on the Canadian market. Exenatide is given by subcutaneous injection prior to breakfast and supper, and helps to lower the glucose levels, particularly after meals. Due to the feedback to the brain satiety center, it allows for improved glucose control with an associated weight loss or at least no weight gain. Because it slows gastric emptying, it can produce nausea, occasional vomiting and some abdominal distension.

*Exenatide*

This medication is given by injection under the skin (subcutaneous) twice a day, before breakfast and supper. It is supplied in pre-filled pens, each containing enough medication for 60 doses. The pens must be kept in the fridge. When used alone, it can be expected to lower A1C by approximately 1 percent. Exanitide can cause:

- mild nausea, especially during the first few weeks of treatment;
- feeling of fullness; or
- weight loss.

| Generic Name | Dose | Contraindications | When to Take It | Comments |
|---|---|---|---|---|
| Exenatide | Usually started with 5 mcg twice daily and may be increased to 10 mcg twice daily if needed. | Renal failure. | 0–60 minutes before breakfast and supper, if forget to take does before the meal, dose should be skipped. | Can cause feeling of fullness and some nausea—usually mild and resolves in a few weeks. |

Pharmaceutical companies are working on various forms of GLP-1-like products, which would have similar effects but do not need to be taken as often. These include liraglutide or exenatide LAR, which may work with 1 injection per day or even per 2–3 weeks.

**DPP-IV Inhibitors (oral medications)**

Another way of obtaining the effects of the GLP-1 would be to enhance the survival of your own GLP-1 by interfering with its natural breakdown. If the enzyme (DPP-IV) that breaks down GLP-1 is blocked, the normally produced GLP-1 effect would be helped. There are now products on the market that do just that and have been shown to improve after-meal glucose control, as do the GLP-1 agonists. Since the amount of GLP-1 is not increased above normal, these medications do not appear to affect the brain's satiety, so weight loss is not seen; however, neither is weight gain even though glucose control improves.

| Generic Name | Dose | Contra-indications | When to Take it | Comments |
|---|---|---|---|---|
| Sitagliptin | Usually begin with 100 mg once daily | Pregnancy | Ideally at a consistent time, either morning or evening, whichever is easier to remember | Occasionally associated with increased rates of minor infection |

Sitagliptin can cause:

- stuffy or runny nose;
- sore throat;
- headache;
- stomach pain;
- diarrhea; and
- very rarely (but serious if occurs), rash or swelling of the face, lips, tongue and throat.

Tell your doctor if any of these symptoms are severe or do not go away.

An underlying concern with this treatment is that the enzyme being blocked is everywhere and affects the breakdown of many other products in the body. This might mean undesirable side effects—of which we are currently unaware—in other systems. Sitagliptin, one formulation of a DPP-IV inhibitor, is on the market and another similar drug called vildagliptin is also marketed in the United States, but not in Canada at the time of printing.

### Pramlintide

Hormones other than insulin are also present in your pancreas, and released in response to food. One of these hormones, "amylin," is produced, stored and secreted in the same way and at the same time as insulin in response to food. This hormone has a role in slowing stomach emptying and decreasing the amount of glucose the liver releases by reducing the effect of glucagon. In addition, amylin sends messages back to the brain when adequate food has been eaten (satiety feedback).

In diabetes, your beta cells not only have difficulty producing enough insulin, but also do not make enough amylin. You cannot give amylin as you do insulin; however, pramlintide is a synthetic molecule that has a similar structure and can be used as a treatment. Pramlintide is approved by the U.S. Food and Drug Administration for use as an additional therapy to help control the rise in glucose after a meal for people with both type 1 and type 2 diabetes who are unable to achieve the desired glucose control. This drug treatment is not recommended for those who have an A1C of more than 9 percent, or who have hypoglycemia unawareness (page 160), eating disorders or gastroparesis (a problem with stomach emptying). In addition, it is felt that people using pramlintide need to check their blood glucose frequently both before and after meals and be prepared to follow up regularly with their doctor. It is not available in Canada at time of printing.

Pramlintide can cause:

- some nausea especially during the first few weeks of treatment;
- hypoglycemia in the initial weeks of therapy before insulin doses are adjusted adequately downward;
- feeling of fullness;
- weight loss of 1–4 kg, related to reduction of appetite.

| Generic Name | Dose | Contra-indications | When to Take it | Comments |
|---|---|---|---|---|
| Pramlintide | Usually started with 15 mcg before meals with at least 30 g of carbohydrates. Can increase by 15 mcg increments to a maximum of 60 mcg before meals if needed | Poor compliance with present insulin and glucose checking regimens, A1C above 9 %, hypoglycemia unawareness, eating disorders or major problems with stomach emptying, pregnancy | Within 15 minutes of the meal. If taken earlier, may help satiety; if taken closer to the meal, may decrease nausea. | Must look for hypoglycemia carefully at initiation of therapy and reduce insulin dose if needed. Nausea often improves with time. |

The expected decrease in A1C from these medications when used alone is 0.5–0.7 percent.

The use of pramlintide is *not* recommended for people with very high A1Cs as at these levels, insulin is too deficient to allow pramlintide to have any positive effect and may make their condition decline.

## Combinations of Medications

As you have seen, each of these groups of medications works in different ways, and so they are often used in combination. Some of the pharmaceutical companies have even started producing combination tablets. This makes it easier for you, as you then have to take only one tablet to get the benefit of two medications. Combination pills available in some countries are metformin and glyburide, metformin and rosiglitazone, metformin and glipizide, and metformin and sitagliptin. Different formulations are available so you can get different doses of each medication. Ask your pharmacist or doctor for details.

### Mary's story

Mary has done well managing her diabetes for several years. She now enjoys her weekly bowling and the aquafitness classes she does twice a week. As well, she has been feeling much better since she has been making healthier choices with her food. Recently, however, the doctor has told her that her blood glucose levels have been creeping up and it is time to add some medication to the management plan. The doctor suggests Mary start with 250 mg of metformin at breakfast and supper. Mary does feel some mild abdominal cramping for the first few days but because the doctor had warned her about this she sticks with it and the cramping goes away. After two weeks her blood glucose results have not improved very much so the doctor suggests she increase to 500 mg twice a day to achieve the target glucose levels they had agreed on. At the higher dose Mary finds her blood glucose levels are mostly in the target range. She contacts her doctor and they decide she should add a midday dose of metformin as well. On this, she finds her glucose levels are now well controlled.

## What Happens If I Miss a Dose?

Medications should be taken at the same time every day and doses should not be skipped. If for some reason you do forget to take your medication, the worst that will happen is that your blood glucose will be higher for a while, until you get it back on track. For most kinds of diabetes medications you can take your missed dose as soon as you remember—as long as it is not too close to your next scheduled dose.

However, if you are taking:

- a sulphonylurea or meglitinide, you should wait until your next meal, as it might cause a low blood glucose if taken between meals;
- acarbose, you should wait for the next meal, as it works only with a meal;
- exenatide, you should wait for the next meal, as it works only with a meal;
- pramlintide, you should wait for the next meal, as it works only with a meal.

### Should I Double up My Dose If I Eat More?

Sometimes you might be tempted to double up on your medication if you know you are going to eat more than usual. This is generally not a good idea because most tablets have fairly long periods of action and might be still working long after your meal has been digested. As well, doubling the number of tablets may not result in double the effect; in fact, the added effect might be minimal. If you are thinking about doubling a dose, speak to your doctor first to ask if it is a good solution. This will partly depend on which medication you are taking. If you know you are going to a party or social event where there will be a lot of food, be sure you do some extra physical activity that day, or at the event, such as dancing.

**If I Skip a Meal, Should I Skip the Medication?**
Of course, ideally you would not skip a meal, but realistically it does happen from time to time. If you do skip a meal you should also skip the medications that directly target the after-meal blood glucose levels, such as repaglinide and nateglinide. For those that cause the pancreas to release more insulin more slowly and over a longer period like the sulphonylureas, it is useful to discuss with your doctor whether or not you should skip a dose when the meal is skipped. Also, acarbose and orlistat should be skipped as they work only when taken directly before the meal.

| If You Skip a Meal... | | |
|---|---|---|
| Skip a Dose | Don't Skip a Dose | Check with Your Doctor |
| acarbose | metformin | glyburide |
| repaglinide | pioglitazone | gliclazide |
| nateglinide | rosiglitazone | glimepiride |
| exenatide | rosiglitazone and metformin combination pill | |
| orlistat | sitagliptin | |
| pramlintide | vidagliptin | |

**What If I Keep Having Low Blood Glucose Levels on My Medication?**
If you find that you are frequently having low blood glucose levels, try to determine the cause:

- Have you reduced your weight?
- Are you keeping to your healthy meal plan more strictly?
- Are you more active than before?

If any of these are the reason, speak to your doctor. You may need less medication. Usually, the medication that pushes your body to release more insulin (sulphonylureas or meglitinides) should be gradually decreased before reducing either the insulin sensitizers (like metformin or the glitazones) or incretin mimetics (like exenatide, stagliptin or vildagliptin).

**Can I Take the Pills When I Get Pregnant?**
Some people who have significant insulin resistance have trouble getting pregnant, and may ovulate better if they are on metformin to decrease the effect of insulin resistance. Metformin has not been shown to be a problem in early pregnancy although the children of these pregnancies have not been followed for the long term, so it is unknown if the metformin has some untoward effect on them in later years. The thiazolidinediones are not recommended during pregnancy as their effect is unknown and sustained usage can cause problems.

When pregnant, it is important for you and your baby that your glucose control be optimal. This will help to prevent birth defects. Prior to conception is the best time to stop the oral diabetes medication and switch to insulin. Once pregnancy is established, it is safest to use insulin, not oral medication. There are rare situations where the use of oral medications might be considered at various points in the pregnancy, but this is best worked out with a diabetes health care team experienced in the management of pregnancy. After the baby is born, there is often a good chance that you can return to the oral medications if they worked prior to pregnancy. If you are breast-feeding, there is some controversy over how safe it is to use either sulphonylureas or metformin since they are minimally detectable in human milk. There are many places in the world where it is considered acceptable to take oral agents while breast-feeding. The use of insulin is not controversial, since it is a hormone normally present. It is important to discuss these issues with your doctor. It is important to plan a future pregnancy, so you should discuss birth control and pregnancy planning with your health care team at this time as well.

Understanding the way your oral medications work will make it easier for you to use them properly. Many medications address the different deficiencies present in type 2 diabetes—those of insulin resistance and decreasing insulin availability. Additional medications that are pharmacological or drug forms of natural gut hormones are now on the market in some countries. However, while these medications facilitate after-meal control in both type 1 and type 2 diabetes, they may have significant side effects. These medications, since they are hormones, can be given only by injection

---

*Remember, the information in this chapter is a basic overview of available medication. You must always discuss starting or changing any medication with your doctor.*

# SEVEN

# Insulin—The "Magic Juice"

I nsulin is a very effective treatment; some people call it the "magic juice," yet almost everyone is hesitant to start it—probably because the only really effective way to give insulin is by injection. Insulin is the missing key for everyone with diabetes: if they didn't lack some insulin production relative to their needs, they would not have diabetes. Coupled with healthy eating and lifestyle, virtually everyone can control diabetes with insulin. People with type 1 diabetes need insulin to live and survive. For those with type 2 diabetes, insulin may be harder to accept, as it is not usually required at diagnosis. However, some insulin might be started with a small dose at night to normalize the pre-breakfast glucose and then healthy eating, exercise and oral medications are able to keep the glucose levels normal all day long.

*Catherine's story*
Catherine is a third-year university student just going into end-of-semester exams. She's been so tired lately that she hasn't been able to go out with her friends after studying. In fact,

studying seems harder—harder to concentrate and occasionally harder to see clearly. The other thing is, she's not sleeping well, having to get up to go to the bathroom so often! After a couple of weeks of this, she finally feels so tired that she's nauseated all the time and actually feels weak. She goes to the campus medical clinic where the physician there checks her capillary glucose and finds it very high—34 mmol/L (612 mg/dl)! Catherine is sent immediately to the emergency room where they do a number of tests, start an intravenous solution, and start her on insulin. The doctors tell her that they think that she has type 1 diabetes. She's very discouraged, but they show her how to take insulin injections, how to check her glucose, and begin to teach her what to eat. Within a day or two, she has regained her energy and feels much better. Within a week, she feels almost as well as she did before she got sick. This insulin business seems to be magic after feeling so exhausted!

## Thomas's story

Thomas has had diabetes now for 15 years. He started with adjustments to what he ate, then his doctor had him take medications that helped him keep his glucose in the target range. Lately, his glucose results have not been good at all. His before-breakfast results are 8–9 mmol/L (144–162 mg/dl). When he checks after meals, which is rare because he doesn't like to see the numbers, the glucose levels are often above 12 mmol/L (216 mg/dl). He takes three different medications for diabetes, some of which cost a lot of money. He just doesn't feel good and he keeps getting annoying little skin infections and boils. The soles of his feet sometimes burn in the night for no reason. His doctor has been suggesting for a while that he start insulin, even if only at night to get his morning glucose corrected. He hesitates ...

Insulin is a hormone with multiple actions that is essential for life as described in Chapters One and Three. Insulin is released from the islets 24 hours a day. Although, if you are not eating, the amount is very low, it is never zero. The automatic release of insulin in response to glucose levels is how blood glucose is kept normal in a person without diabetes. In diabetes the goal is to match available insulin to the way insulin was released before diabetes developed.

## Where Does the Insulin Used to Treat Diabetes Come From?

**Early Years**
Originally, when Frederick Banting and Charles Best first isolated insulin, it was prepared using either beef or pork pancreata that were broken down and the insulin in them purified. Amino acids are the building blocks that make up proteins like insulin in our bodies. Beef insulin is different from our own insulin by three amino acids and pork insulin is different by only one. The earliest insulin had many impurities and often produced problems, such as swelling and rashes at the injection sites. In the 1970s, the ability to purify the insulin was dramatically improved so that the problems previously seen at injection sites have almost disappeared.

The purified insulin was combined with zinc as a crystal and kept in a buffered solution so that it would stay active when kept in a refrigerator for one to two years. This insulin was like human insulin and worked quickly when injected, but once injected, it didn't last very long. It was called "regular" or soluble insulin. This kind of insulin had to be given at least three or four times a day in order to ensure some insulin was available at all times.

In the 1940s, a Danish scientist named Hagedorn discovered a way to add a fish protein, protamine, to insulin, which allowed it to be released from its crystal much more slowly after injection. This insulin was called Neutral Protamine Hagedorn insulin, now called NPH or N insulin. Not long after that, it was discovered that adding more zinc to the insulin crystal further stabilized it after an injection and made it act more slowly. These kinds of insulin are called Lente and Ultralente insulins. The prolongation of the action of these insulins allowed them to be used two or three times a day or, in some cases, where the insulin lack was less severe, even once a day.

### Human Insulin Formulations

In the 1970s and early 1980s, technology developed that allowed the gene from the human insulin molecule to be inserted inside other cells that would then make human insulin. These products were then purified and combined with zinc in a crystal. The Lilly insulin company used a kind of simple bacterial cell (*Escherichia coli*), which reproduces rapidly, to act as the carrier for the human insulin gene and make large amounts of human insulin. The Novo-Nordisk insulin company did the same thing but used baker's yeast to make the human insulin molecules. These insulins take about 20 to 30 minutes to start acting and in most people, last about 6 to 8 hours. They are often referred to as "short-" or "fast-" acting insulins. The original product produced as human insulin was equivalent to soluble or regular insulin purified from pancreata of pigs, but with the same amino acids as we make in our bodies. In order to provide slower absorption of the insulin, this purified human insulin molecule was combined with protamine or with increased amounts of zinc.

## Insulins Made for Specific Purposes: "Designer" or "Analogue" Insulins

More recently, as the specifics of how insulin acts have been better understood, insulin analogues have been developed. These insulins have been called "designer" insulins because they were created by design for specific purposes.

### Rapid-acting analogues

Normally insulin is stored as a crystal with a molecule of zinc in the middle and six molecules of insulin attached around. When insulin is released into your blood, the molecules (called monomers) separate from the zinc and go in the blood to the various cells where they act.

To form rapid-acting insulin, the insulin has been changed where it connects with zinc so that the monomers of insulin do not form a stable crystal, but prefer to be separate. Once the insulin is injected under the skin, the time for it to dissociate or separate into individual parts is much faster. This is how rapid-acting insulin analogues can act within 10 to 15 minutes of injection. Their peak action is at about 1 to 1 1/2 hours after injection and by 4 to 5 hours later, in most people, there are minimal amounts left in the blood. The short action times of rapid-acting analogues allows their use in individualized regimens.

### Slower-acting basal analogues

Insulin has been altered to slow it in other ways. Insulin glargine is liquid but, at the pH level under the skin, it forms a crystal that dissolves very slowly. Insulin detemir has a prolonged duration of action because the insulin has been adjusted to combine with a natural protein in the blood (albumin). The insulin then circulates in your blood, being released only slowly from this molecule.

All these insulin formulations have made it progressively easier to reproduce the normal physiology of insulin in our bodies and keep glucose levels normal.

---

## Insulin formulations

- **Soluble, short acting or regular (R) insulin** is equivalent to human insulin. It exists in solution as a crystal with eight individual molecules of insulin (monomers) around a zinc molecule. Once given subcutaneously, it is dissolved in the fluid under the skin and the crystal dissociates to the individual monomers, which are absorbed.

- **Rapid-acting analogue insulins** decrease the connection to zinc so crystals are not formed or are less stable. They have a faster dissociation in subcutaneous tissue: lispro, aspart, glulisine.

- **Insulin formulations with slower actions** lengthen the time for the dissociation of the insulin crystal to occur by:
  - addition of protamine (a fish protein): NPH;
  - higher zinc concentration: Lente insulins;
  - changes of pH-creating crystals under the skin: glargine;
  - binding to albumin enhanced: detemir.

---

## Inhaled Insulins

Inhaled insulin was on the market for a short time in the United States, but was withdrawn. Since other companies may bring inhaled insulin to market, the basic concepts are covered here. The insulin is regular insulin that has been attached to a medium or substance that can help carry the insulin molecule into your lungs when you take a breath. To take a dose, the person activates the insulin delivery device, releasing the insulin "powder" or solution into the aerosol chamber while taking a deep breath—like using an inhaler for asthma. The insulin is carried into the lungs and passed into the capillaries very quickly. The peak effect of inhaled insulin was as fast as or faster than the rapid-acting analog insulins like lispro or aspart.

Interestingly, the duration of action appeared to be a bit longer, more like "regular" insulin.

If insulin can be inhaled and doesn't need an injection, why doesn't everyone take it that way? Maybe one day this will be a popular option for insulin delivery, but currently there are some disadvantages and concerns.

- Inhaled insulin is only rapid-acting insulin. In order to cover the background insulin needs for day and the night, it is still necessary for people to inject a longer-acting insulin.
- Huge amounts of insulin are needed to be combined with the carrier protein to deliver enough insulin to the blood-stream to work—about eight times as much, which raises the cost considerably.
- Many people who used the marketed form of insulin developed a dry cough. Although it improves with time, it might persist in some.
- In some patients, especially those with type 1 diabetes, there are antibodies formed against insulin, as was seen with the impure insulins used in the 1970s and before. The importance of this is unknown.
- As yet, it is not clear what effect smoking will have on the inhaled insulin.
- Insulin is a growth factor (stimulates the growth of cells), which is now being delivered directly to the lung. As yet, we do not know if or how inhaling insulin might have an impact on the risks for lung cancer or breathing abnormalities after years of use.

Other companies are working toward other inhaler devices that would use a liquid insulin formulation rather than a powder. Experiments are also being done with the potential for orally active insulin that would be absorbed by the tissues lining the mouth cavity.

# How Do We "Marry" the Food Peak with the Insulin Peak?

Now that you know the basic forms of insulin available, how do you combine them so that the insulin is "there" at the surface of the cell when the glucose from the food arrives? To be effective, the two must coincide closely for the insulin to help the cell access the glucose from the blood and use that glucose to make energy.

For insulin to match your needs perfectly, there would have to be a constant small amount (to cover *basal* needs) and a little extra (a *bolus*) each time you eat. The method of injection that most closely reproduces this is an insulin pump, where tiny amounts of baseline or basal insulin are given throughout the day and, whenever food is eaten, an appropriate amount of insulin (the rapid analogue kind) is given as a bolus. This method of delivery is very expensive and, for most people who need insulin, this degree of precise delivery is not needed. The idea of the pump, however, conveys the concept of how to try to take insulin, that is, the idea of basal and bolus needs.

# Who Needs to Take Insulin for Treatment?

## Type 2 Diabetes

If you have type 2 diabetes and control your glucose values by:

*Healthy eating and physical activity alone ...*
This means that you are able to keep your blood glucose values, especially the fasting glucose levels, in the target range by following a healthy meal plan and doing regular physical activity. In most situations, unless demands are very great due to severe stress or illness, you have adequate basal and bolus insulin.

*Healthy eating, physical activity, and oral medications ...*
This means that you are able to, with the help of either insulin

sensitizers or insulin-stimulating medications, make enough insulin for most daily life situations. However, illness, pregnancy, or times of prolonged stress can result in high glucose levels. Temporary administration of insulin at these times will keep glucose levels within range. Once the stress is resolved, glucose levels can again be controlled by oral medications.

*Healthy eating, physical activity with or without glucose-lowering medications, but requiring insulin ...*
This means that you are unable to keep your glucose levels within target range with healthy eating, activity, and medications, other than insulin, under normal life situations. Even without the additional stresses of illness, you need insulin to keep your glucose within the target range. In times of illness or stresses, you are likely to need more insulin.

With the passage of time, cells that produce insulin are lost, a natural process of aging like hair going whiter. People with type 2 diabetes already didn't have enough insulin, so as the amount of available insulin decreases; they may not have enough insulin for their needs and eventually must take it to feel well. If you are overweight when you get diabetes, you don't have enough insulin for your needs but you are still able to make a lot of insulin. Successful weight loss may allow you to manage a long time on the insulin that you have in reserve, If you are normal weight when you are diagnosed with type 2 diabetes, you have less reserve ability to make insulin and, with loss of your body's insulin reserves over time, you may actually need help with injections of insulin before those who are obese. In fact, some people who appear to have type 2 diabetes initially will eventually have as severe an insulin deficiency as a person with type 1 diabetes.

### Type 1 Diabetes

If you have type 1 diabetes, you need insulin to live, since you have virtually no beta cells left to make insulin. After starting insulin and achieving blood glucose levels in the target range, you may experience what is termed a "honeymoon" phase. This usually occurs within one to three months after treatment starts. The beta cells that were damaged but not destroyed have been given a rest while you have been injecting insulin, and some of the inflammation around them may decrease. This can result in some production of insulin again, which might mean that you can reduce the amount of injected insulin, sometimes down to almost nothing. Although it might seem like a good idea to stop insulin completely, this is not usually recommended as it has been shown that optimal blood glucose levels will prolong the life of the remaining beta cells. Unfortunately, this "honeymoon" phase does not last forever—usually only from a few months to 18 months. The longer that your beta cells continue to produce any insulin the better, since this will help decrease the ups and downs of controlling the glucose. The older you are when diagnosed with type 1 diabetes, the longer it usually takes for the remaining beta cells to cease to function—anywhere from 5 to 10 years. After this point, glucose control may become more difficult, with more swings of glucose seen.

## Getting Started with Insulin

If your doctor has told you that you need insulin, there are a number of things you need to learn prior to starting. Ideally, your doctor, diabetes nurse educator, and dietitian (in a diabetes teaching center) will help you learn the answers to these questions:

- How and when do the insulins you take work?
- When do you need to take the insulin in relation to food and time of day?
- Should your eating patterns be adjusted when starting insulin?
- How would you treat hypoglycemia (see also Chapter Eight)?
- How do you prepare and give the insulin injection?
- How do you store and care for your insulin supplies?
- How do you monitor your blood glucose (see also Chapter Five)?
- How do you interpret your blood glucose results (see also Chapters Five and Eight)?
- How do you adjust your dose of insulin, if appropriate (see also Chapters Five and Eight)?

**How and When Do the Insulins You Take Work?**
As discussed in the first part of this chapter, there are many different types of insulin. Not all types of insulin are available in all countries. Always know the name of the insulin you are taking, how long it takes to start to work, and how long it lasts. In Canada, insulin is sold only as 100 units per mL (U100). In some parts of the world, there are other concentrations sold such as 40 units per mL (U40) or 80 units per mL (U80). It is very important that you use the syringe that matches the type of insulin you are using. That is, if using 40 unit/ml insulin you must have a syringe calibrated to 40 units/ml so your dose remains the same.

Internationally, the labels on insulin vials or cartridges have been color coded so that no matter where you are, you should know what type of insulin you are buying. Refer to the International Diabetes Federation Web site to see the insulin color codes (www.idf.org).

Remember that insulins work differently in different people

and can even work differently in the same person on different days.

| | Name | Approximate Time to Start | Approximate Peak Action | Approximate Duration |
|---|---|---|---|---|
| Rapid-acting analogues | Apidra–glusine Humalog–lispro NovoRapid–aspart | 10–15 minutes | 60–90 minutes | 3–5 hours |
| Short-acting (soluble) | Humulin R–regular Novolin ge Toronto or R–regular Hypurin Regular (pork) | 30–60 minutes | 2–4 hours | 5–8 hours |
| Inter-mediate-acting | Humulin N-NPH Novolin ge NPH Lente* Hypurin NPH (pork) | 1–3 hours | 5–8 hours | Up to 18 hours |
| Long-acting | Ultralente* | 3–4 hours | 8–15 hours | 22–26 hours |
| Extended long-acting analogue | Lantus–glargine Novolin Levemir-detemir | 90 minutes | No peak | 22–26 hours 16–24 hours dependant on dose |
| Premixed regular insulin and NPH | Humulin 30/70, Novolin ge 30/70, 40/60, 50/50 | The time action is related to the amount of each insulin that is in the mix. In Canada, the first number in the premix indicates the percent of short- or rapid-acting insulin. The second number is the percent of intermediate-acting insulin. In the United States, the numbers are reversed. | | |
| Premixed insulin analogues | Humalog Mix25 and Mix 50–inuslin lispro/ lispro protamine mix NovoMix30–biphasic insulin aspart | | | |

*No longer available in Canada.
Note: This is not an exhaustive list of available insulins in all parts of the world.

Conditions that will affect how your insulins work are:
- The injection site—insulin is absorbed fastest from the abdomen, then the upper arms, outer thighs, and buttocks. The site used is less important with the rapid-acting analogue insulins.
- The temperature of the insulin—insulin at room temperature is absorbed faster than insulin right out of the fridge.
- The temperature of the skin—if the area of injection is

warm, as on a hot day, after exercise or rubbing the skin, insulin will be absorbed faster.

- The angle of injection—insulin should be injected between 45 and 90 degrees. If the angle of injection is too shallow, absorption will be slower.
- The amount of adipose tissue (fat)—insulin will be absorbed faster when there is less adipose tissue.
- The volume of insulin injected—the higher the dose, the slower the absorption. Some recommend that if your dose is more than 50 units, you split it into two and give two injections.
- If the skin has become thickened due to repeated use of the same injection site, absorption at these sites is much less reliable.

Many years ago, when insulin was not as pure, an abnormality called lipodystrophy was seen at the sites of injection. The skin appeared to have either caved in or formed a bump. This is rarely seen now that purer insulins are available, but if you have developed a bump, avoid injecting into that area as the insulin will not be absorbed as well, or at least inject around the outside rather than repeatedly in the same spot.

### When Do You Need to Take the Insulin in Relation to Food and Time of Day?

You, your doctor, and your diabetes health care team will work out the best routine for you. There are many, many ways of using insulin to control blood glucose. It is said that if you ask 10 different endocrinologists (doctors who treat conditions of the endocrine glands and hormones) what regimen to use, you would get 10 different answers. The best regimen is the one that works best for you.

If you use regular/soluble insulin, ideally, it should be taken about 30 minutes prior to eating, so that it will be absorbed in time for the glucose peak of the meal. If your glucose is very low before starting a meal, treat the low (see Chapter Eight: hypoglycemia) to increase your glucose level before taking the insulin for your meal. If your glucose is low, it may be safer not to delay the meal for more than 15 minutes. Conversely, if your glucose is very high prior to eating a meal, it may help to delay the meal by 15 to 20 more minutes, thereby allowing the glucose to come closer to normal levels prior to eating. Many people find the use of the rapid-acting analogues easier, since they can be taken just as you begin to eat, ideally 5 to 15 minutes before. However, if you forgot or weren't sure how much you would eat, they still work quite well if taken up to 15 minutes after starting the meal.

> Thomas is getting more and more worried, and tired, since his morning glucose keeps going higher and higher and he doesn't even check after meals because it frightens him. He finally accepts his doctors' suggestion to start NPH insulin before bedtime. The dietitian suggests that he move a small amount of starch and protein from his lunch meal to just before bedtime at around the same time that he takes the insulin. He starts with 8 units of insulin the first night. He succeeds in taking it! The only thing is, his glucose level the next day is still above 9 mmol/L (162 mg/dl). Following his doctor's recommendation, he gradually increases the dose by 1 to 2 units every 2 to 4 days until he starts seeing morning glucose levels below 7 mmol/L (126 mg/dl). Incredibly, the rest of his glucose levels in the day start to look much better and he feels much more energetic! Why did he wait so long? This insulin business isn't that big a deal!

The following are some of the most commonly used regimens, but many variations are possible:

*Overnight insulin*

- For many people with type 2 diabetes, a dose of intermediate (NPH) insulin at bedtime or long acting (glargine or
detemir) insulin at supper or bedtime is all that is needed
to achieve target pre-breakfast glucose levels. You will
usually start with a relatively low amount and slowly
increase the amount until the fasting glucose is in the target
range you and your doctor have chosen. Because you will
feel so much better once your glucose levels are within the
target range, you may be inspired to increase your activity or improve your eating habits. This may lower your
blood glucose, possibly too low. Should this happen, your
insulin dose needs to be lowered. Many doctors will
include a lower number in the target, so if your glucose
goes below that, you can reduce the dose by 1 to 2 units.
If your dose is not lowered, you might feel a need to "eat
up to your dose," which can result in weight gain.
- Working with your doctor and/or nurse educator, you
can look at *patterns* in your blood glucose results and
make adjustments. For example, if your blood glucose
value in the morning (before eating) is consistently low
(under 4–5 mmol/L (72–90 mg/dl), it might be appropriate to reduce the evening dose of insulin to raise your
morning level a little. On the other hand, you may be following your meal plan, yet your morning glucose level is
always high. In this case, your insulin might need to be
slightly increased.
- The cells that make insulin are unable to work well if sur-
rounded by excess glucose. This is called "glucose toxic-
ity." Using overnight insulin to improve the glucose level
at the beginning of the day allows the beta cells to release
more insulin, so your efforts at healthy eating and activity
and the working of your other diabetes medications are

more effective. You may even need to decrease their doses.
- Over time, the advantage obtained by normalizing the fasting glucose level using overnight insulin might not be enough to allow your islet cells to work throughout the day. They gradually lose the ability to release insulin in response to the normal stimuli of a meal. At this point, additional doses of insulin could be needed.

*Insulin before breakfast and to cover the night*
- When overnight insulin alone is no longer effective, you will need to add insulin in the morning. This might be an intermediate-acting insulin that is given to try to decrease glucose levels during the day. However, because it takes a couple of hours for intermediate-acting insulin to work, this approach can result in high blood glucose results after breakfast and before lunch. Most people would also take a shorter-acting insulin (either regular/soluble or a rapid-acting analogue) with the morning intermediate insulin.
- One way to take the two types of insulin would be to use a "premixed" insulin. Premixed insulins are combinations of regular/soluble or rapid-acting insulin combined with intermediate-acting insulin. In Canada, the first number is the percentage of regular/soluble or rapid-acting, the second number the percentage of intermediate-acting insulin. In some countries (for example, the United States) the numbers are reversed so that the percentage of intermediate-acting insulin is first.

Example:
- In Canada: 30/70 means 30 percent regular insulin, 70 percent intermediate-acting insulin.
- In the U.S.: 70/30 means the same thing.

*Insulin before breakfast and supper, and for overnight*
Adding insulin in the morning will often successfully correct the morning and afternoon blood glucose levels, but rarely will it correct blood glucose levels in the period *after* supper. Supper is often the main meal of the day and a time when a lot of glucose-containing food is ingested. With insulin taken before breakfast and for overnight only, your glucose results after supper and in the evening might be too high. In order to have adequate insulin to cover the glucose from your supper meal, you might need to add either regular/soluble or a rapid-acting analogue prior to eating that meal. Many people can get excellent control for long periods of time using a regimen like this.

*Insulin before breakfast and before supper*
As a compromise to taking insulin three times a day, glucose control in some people with type 2 diabetes can be achieved using insulin twice a day—before breakfast and before supper. In this situation, regular/soluble or a rapid-acting analogue is given with an intermediate or long-acting insulin. A common combination is a 30/70 pre-mix prior to breakfast and a 50/50 premix before supper. There are innumerable possibilities for these mixes and finding the one that is right for you is best worked out with your diabetes team, using the results of your blood glucose checking. The potential difficulty of using an intermediate-acting insulin at supper is that it begins to peak about five to eight hours after it is taken, which for people who eat around 6 PM is between 11 PM and 3 AM. For this reason, this regimen usually requires a meal plan adjustment to ensure that you eat a snack before bedtime to prevent nighttime hypoglycemia during the peak action hours.

*Insulin before meals and bedtime*
For people with type 1 and those with type 2 diabetes who have

very little to no insulin of their own, the safest insulin regimen to use is regular or rapid-acting insulin prior to each meal and an intermediate or long-acting insulin to provide the background basal and night coverage. The overnight control of glucose is essential to start the day with a good glucose level.

• This type of routine works particularly well for people who work shifts or whose meals are at different times on different days. For instance, if you have a very long afternoon, that is, an early lunch and late supper, using only the rapid-acting analogue at lunch might cover only half your afternoon. Another small injection of the rapid-acting analogue mid-afternoon with a snack may be the answer, or the use of regular/soluble insulin at lunch with a lower carbohydrate load at lunch and a mid-afternoon snack could work better. Insulin patterns can, and should, be individualized to meet your needs. Discuss with your doctor or diabetes educator how best to change your insulin patterns to meet your needs.

## Insulin Infusion Pumps

Pumps are the method of insulin delivery that comes closest to the body's own actions. Used effectively, pumps allow most people to achieve near-normal glucose levels, although not without significant effort. In individuals, particularly with type 1 diabetes, where the control of the overnight glucose levels is highly variable and/or they have big variations in glucose values from high to low, the use of an insulin pump could be the only way to successfully control their diabetes. Over the years, they have become substantially more sophisticated and, although still very expensive, have gradually become a mainstream form of therapy in type 1 diabetes.

If you are on a pump, your insulin is delivered through a small catheter that you place under the skin of your abdomen or upper thigh. A continuous amount of "basal" insulin is delivered over 24 hours. The amount is tailored to your individual activity level, body size, and precise insulin needs. Once the basal is correctly established, the glucose levels should stay within a normal range whether you eat or not.

When you do eat, you decide on the amount of bolus insulin required. The factors that you need to consider will be your present glucose level, exactly what foods you plan to eat (ideally with a guesstimate of the amount of carbohydrate content) and the activities that you expect to be doing while that dose of insulin is acting. You would key this amount as "bolus" and activate. The insulin can be delivered all at once, similar to an injection of insulin with a needle, or in small amounts or waves to better match the type of meal. Some newer pumps have adaptations that help you do the math to establish the dose of insulin needed. With help from your doctor or diabetes health care team, you will establish the best ratio of units of insulin to the amount of carbohydrate that you eat for each meal. There are many insulin pumps on the market. There is now a pump available with no tubing connections—the pump is attached to the surface of the skin and there is a controller which looks like a cell phone that is used to adjust rates and bolus doses. For pump therapy of any kind to work effectively, a significant amount of learning, is required. Initiation of pump therapy should not be undertaken other than in pump specialty centers.

Catherine is feeling much more comfortable about her diabetes management as the school year winds down. This summer, however, she has plans to take a summer job planting trees and wants to discuss with her doctor whether she needs to change her regimen. Her doctor reminds her that an overall increase in activity will likely result in a decreased need for insulin. As she begins her summer job, she should expect to decrease both her basal insulin and the amount of insulin that she needs for her carbohydrate in the meal. As well, she will have breakfast earlier than usual and lunch may be smaller and later. Her doctor suggests using a small amount of intermediate insulin in addition to her rapid-acting insulin that she uses to cover her breakfast, so that she has background insulin until her later lunch. Catherine is starting to understand that her insulin dose needs to be adapted to any changes in her life and her habits.

## Changing Doses

Once a dose is established, it will rarely stay the same forever. Changes in your weight, activities that are seasonal, enthusiasm for exercise programs that wax and wane, stresses of life or illness, and simply aging can affect your insulin dose and might make adjustments necessary. Many of these issues are reviewed in Chapter Eight.

### Should Your Eating Pattern Be Adjusted When Starting Insulin?

To some degree, the answer will depend on whether you have type 1 or type 2 diabetes. Most importantly, determine how much food you need to have a healthy, nutritious meal plan and how to distribute it throughout the day so that the insulin you take can keep your glucose levels within the target range. A diabetes meal plan can be as simple as eating three meals a day or be as complex as counting carbohydrates and determining an insulin:carbohydrate ratio to decide how much insulin to take at each meal. As with insulin regimens there are many, many plans for healthy eating. A registered dietitian is the best person to help you decide on the best meal plan for you. Every effort should be made to have an individual consultation with a dietitian as soon as possible after the diagnosis of diabetes is made.

**How Do You Prepare and Give the Insulin Injection?**
Whenever possible, your diabetes educator, in consultation with your doctor, will help you decide the best method for your needs. Some pharmacists might be able to help you learn about the ways to inject insulin. There are three methods you can use to inject insulin. Some insulin requires that you use a syringe; most are available in cartridge form and can therefore be used in pens.

*Pens and insulin cartridges*
Insulin for use with insulin pens comes in 3.0 mL (300 units) cartridges. Pens look similar to a fat ballpoint pen. An insulin cartridge is loaded into the pen and a needle placed on the end. A dial at the end of the pen is used to select the dose. Insulin is injected by pushing the plunger.

| Advantages | Disadvantages |
|---|---|
| • Pens are easy to use.<br>• The dose is accurate.<br>• Pens are more discreet than vials and syringes.<br>• Reusing the pen is environmentally friendly. | • A cartridge contains either one kind of insulin or a set premix.<br>• You will need a pen for each type of insulin you use.<br>• You must load cartridges into pens.<br>• You can use a maximum of 60–80 units in one injection, depending on the pen you use. |

When starting to use a pen, refer to the instructions provided. Pens from different manufacturers differ. You should never try to use a cartridge from one company in a pen from another company. Cartridges are designed to fit specific pens and might break or leak if put in different pens.

*Vials and syringes*
A vial is a glass bottle that contains 10 mL (1000 units) of insulin. To use insulin from a vial, you need a syringe. Most people use

two kinds of insulin and therefore have two vials. You could use two syringes and inject twice or, depending on the insulin, it may be possible to put both kinds of insulin into one syringe so you have to inject only once.

| Advantages | Disadvantages |
|---|---|
| • You can vary the amount of each kind of insulin in one injection.<br>• You can give up to 100 units in a single injection, although this might not be recommended. | • It is not discreet to prepare the syringe in public.<br>• Mixing two kinds of insulin in one syringe may be tricky for some people.<br>• There is more room for error getting the exact dose. |

### Pre-filled pens (disposable pens)

Some pens come pre-filled with 3.0 mL (300 units) of a specific type of insulin. When you have used the insulin in these pens you throw them away or recycle them at your pharmacy.

| Advantages | Disadvantages |
|---|---|
| • The pen is easy to use.<br>• The dose is accurate.<br>• The pen is ready to go; there is no cartridge to load.<br>• The pen is more discreet than vials and syringes. | • A pen contains either one kind of insulin or a set premix.<br>• You will need a pen for each type of insulin you use.<br>• Pre-filled pens are more expensive and wasteful.<br>• You can give a maximum of 60–80 units in one injection depending on the pen you use. |

**Preparing a single dose using a vial and syringe:**
Collect the things you need for your injection: the syringe, the vial of insulin, and an alcohol swab.

1. Wash your hands.
2. If using cloudy insulin, gently shake and roll the vial several times to mix it. Vigorous shaking is not recommended. Remove the cap (if the vial is new) and wipe the top of the vial with an alcohol swab.

3. Remove the cap(s) from the syringe and pull back the plunger to the amount of insulin you will be using. This will put air into your syringe equal to your insulin dose.
4. Insert the needle into the vial and inject the air in the syringe into the vial.
5. Without removing the syringe from the vial, turn it upside down and withdraw the units of insulin you require.
6. With the needle still in the vial, look at the syringe to see if there are any air bubbles. If there are, gently tap the syringe so they float to the top, or inject the insulin back into the vial and withdraw again to reach the amount in step 5.
7. Put the vial back on the table and remove the needle from the vial.

The reason for injecting air into the vial is to replace the insulin you will be removing. Because insulin vials are vacuum packed, if you did not put air in, it would become more and more difficult to pull the insulin out.

Although it is advised to try to remove the bubbles from the syringe, if you inject a tiny bubble of air into your body, it will not hurt you. You are injecting into fatty tissue and the bubble will be absorbed. However, you may get less insulin if the bubble is taking up too much space in the syringe.

**Preparing a mixed dose using vials and a syringe:**
If you want to mix two insulins into the same syringe there is a slightly different technique. Note: *You must not mix glargine/Lantus or detemir/Levemir with any other insulin.*

First collect your supplies: a syringe, two vials, and an alcohol swab. It is a good idea to write down how much of each type of insulin you will be using.

1. Wash your hands.

2. Gently shake and roll the cloudy insulin several times to mix it. Wipe the top of the vials with an alcohol swab.
3. Remove the cap(s) from the syringe and pull back the plunger to the amount of cloudy insulin you will be using.
4. Insert the needle into the cloudy insulin vial and inject the air in the syringe into the vial.
5. Remove the empty syringe from the vial.
6. Pull back on the plunger to the amount of clear insulin you will be using.
7. Insert the needle into the clear insulin vial and inject this air into the vial.
8. Without removing the syringe from the vial, turn it upside down and withdraw the amount of clear insulin you need. Look at the syringe to see if there are any air bubbles. If there are, tap the syringe so they float to the top or inject the insulin back into the vial and withdraw insulin again.
9. Now put the needle into the cloudy insulin vial, turn it upside down and withdraw the amount of cloudy insulin you need to make up your total dose.
10. Remove the needle from the vial and check for bubbles. If you have bubbles this time you cannot put the insulin back into the vial, but must simply tap the syringe and hope they float to the top so you can push them into the air.

Be careful not to inject any clear insulin into the cloudy vial; if you do, the cloudy vial should be discarded. If you withdraw too much insulin from the cloudy vial, you should probably discard that dose and start again.

Some people prefer to draw the cloudy insulin into the syringe before the clear insulin. In fact, it really does not matter which you do first, but preparing your injection the same way every day will help you to develop a habit that should reduce the chance of errors.

**Injecting:**

1. Choose a site for injection. As can be seen in the illustration, there are numerous sites that can be used: abdomen, upper arms, outer thighs and buttocks. Some people use only the abdomen for injecting as this results in more consistent absorption. Rotating your sites is important; keep your injection sites about 2.5 cm (1") apart. Some people like to wipe the site with alcohol. This is optional. If you do use alcohol, be sure to let it dry before injecting.

Sites for injection

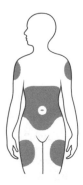

2. Gently pinch up 2.5 cm (1") of fat. If you have a lot of fat in the area chosen you do not have to pinch.
3. Inject the needle straight into the fat, at a 45 to 90 degree angle. You can inject quickly like a dart or slowly push it in, whichever you are comfortable with.
4. Push the plunger all the way down. Release the skin (if pinched) and count to five to minimize leakage.
5. Remove the needle.
   - If you are using one of the shorter needles you may not require "pinching" at the injection site.
   - If you are using a pen or a pre-filled pen, make sure you *push* the plunger, not twist it, when injecting.
   - After finishing the injection, the indicator on the pen should be at "0" or the syringe should be empty.

- Although not necessary, after removal of the needle, a clean dry Kleenex or cotton swab can be held against the site with gentle pressure for 30 to 60 seconds.

Sometimes, after withdrawing the needle, a drop of blood may come out or a small bruise will develop. This is not a concern, but you may have punctured a tiny capillary blood vessel.

**How Do You store and Care for Your Insulin Supplies?**

**Storing your insulin**
The insulin you are using can be kept in the fridge or at room temperature. You may feel the injection less if the insulin is at room temperature, rather than cold from the fridge. Once you have started using the insulin vial or cartridge, most insulin is good for only 28 days. After 28 days, the insulin might not work as well, so even if there is insulin left in the vial, it should be discarded. Always check the manufacturer's information for details on when insulin should be discarded.

Unopened vials, cartridges, and pre-filled pens should be kept in the fridge at 2°C to 8°C (36°F to 46°F). They are good until the expiry date printed on the side of the label. Do not use them after the expiry date.

Insulin is a protein like the white of an egg. If the white of an egg becomes too hot or too cold, it whitens—the protein changes form. When insulin changes its form, it doesn't work. This is why it is important to keep your insulin away from extreme hot or cold temperatures. For example, insulin should never sit in direct sunlight or be placed directly on a freezer pack. If you have to keep it in a car or outside for a period in the summer or winter, you should put it in a small thermos or cooler that will keep it at a constant temperature. It is best to keep your insulin in a temperature range of 2°C to 25°C (36°F to 86°F).

Reusable insulin pens should not be kept in the fridge. The extra, unopened cartridges should be kept in the fridge.

## Checking your insulin

Always look at your insulin before you use it. The clear insulin should always appear clear and colorless. It should not have anything floating in it.

Cloudy insulin may separate when sitting for a period, but it should mix up when you gently shake and roll it several times (when using vials). Cartridges should be gently shaken 10 times and rolled ten times to ensure mixing.

Do not use cloudy insulin if:

- white clumps form that do not dissolve;
- a frosted look is on the vial as if some powder has stuck to the sides;
- powder that will not mix forms at the bottom or around the neck of the vial or cartridge.

### What kinds of syringes are there?

Syringes come in many sizes. Use the syringe that is best suited for your dose. For instance, if your total dose is 35 units, use a 0.50 mL syringe. Available sizes: 0.25 mL, 0.30 mL, 0.50 mL, are 1.00 mL capacity (in other words, 25, 30, 50, or 100 units).

Needles also come in various sizes. The gauge of the needle measures the thickness (29 to 32, higher numbers being thinner) and lengths range from 5 mm to 12.7 mm. A child or a very thin adult would usually use shorter lengths. You might want to use the thinnest, shortest available but you need to check that you are getting effective administration of the insulin. Shorter needles need to be injected at a 90 degree angle to avoid the insulin being injected into the layers of skin instead of into the fat under the skin. An injection intracutaneously (into the skin layer) will hurt as that is where the nerve endings are. Checking your blood glucose levels will help you to determine if you are getting adequate absorption.

## How do I dispose of the needles?

Insulin syringes and needles should never be simply placed in the garbage as they may cause accidental injury to the person who empties the garbage. They should be discarded in a plastic container, such as a shampoo or bleach bottle or a specific container supplied by some pharmacies. Do not dispose of them in a glass container. Some recycling centers will accept used syringes in plastic containers. Ask your pharmacist or diabetes educator for disposal recommendations in your area.

## Can I reuse a needle or syringe?

Health Canada and most health care professionals strongly recommend that syringes and needle tips be used only once. For your personal health and safety, reuse needles only if:

- The needle has not touched anything but your skin and the vial.
- You recap the syringe between uses.
- You have good personal hygiene.
- You do not have other illnesses that might increase your risk of infection.
- The needle is not bent or otherwise damaged.
- The needle was not used by someone else.

If you do choose to use your syringe or needle again, do not wipe the needle with alcohol between uses as doing so may remove the non-stick coating on the needle that makes the injection more comfortable. Use of the needle can cause some minor damage to the sharpness, which if reused, would potentially increase the discomfort.

If you are using a pen or pre-filled pen, it is advised that you remove the needle after completion of each injection. Do not store the pen with the needle attached. Removing the needle will help ensure sterility and prevent leakage, re-entry of air, and potential needle clogs.

Using insulin might seem scary at first, but once you know how to safely inject, you will find it routine. Insulin really is "the magic juice" as it will make you feel so much better and healthier when used correctly. Remember, your need for insulin will change over time and as your lifestyle changes; be sure to keep in contact with your doctor and health care team to keep your management plan up to date.

# EIGHT

# Highs, Lows, and Adjustments

Hyperglycemia or high blood glucose levels even slightly above target can increase the risk of complications related to diabetes. Glucose levels that are either very high for a few years or persistently a little high for many years increase the risks of developing "chronic" or long-term complications—the degree of accumulated "extra" glucose seems to lead to problems. This chapter will discuss the acute complications. Chapter Nine will discuss the chronic complications. Acute conditions develop quickly and may resolve fairly quickly. Chronic conditions usually take time to develop and persist over time.

### David's story

David is an accountant and likes to be precise. Although 50 pounds (23 kg) overweight with a pretty good "beer belly," he pays attention to his personal care and feels that he takes care of himself. Lately, he has had annoying skin irritations in his groin and now he has a nasty boil on his buttock. He goes to his family doctor who gives him a cream for his rash, drains his boil and sends him to the lab to check his blood glucose level. The doctor calls David to tell him his glucose level is 15.3 mmol/L (275 mg/dl)! He puts him on tablets to lower his blood glucose and makes sure that David gets an appointment at the diabetes center. David takes his diet seriously and begins his medications. Before long, his glucose levels are under 6 mmol/L (108 mg/dl) most mornings. When he checks his glucose after breakfast or supper, it's between 6 and 7.5 mmol/L (108 and 135 mg/dl) instead of 16 (288) as it was before. His skin infections have cleared up and he feels much better.

We will follow David's activities throughout this chapter.

## The Highs: Acute Complications of Hyperglycemia

Everyone with diabetes will have high glucose levels from time to time but the key is to minimize the length of time you spend above your target level. Mild persistent elevations of glucose can often lead to annoying small infections and increased frequency of infections. When the glucose is elevated, the risk of more serious infections increases and the stress caused by these infections pushes the glucose levels even higher. A vicious cycle!

### Problems with Infections

Generally, people with diabetes do not have difficulty treating infections or recurrent infections unless they have uncontrolled diabetes. When diabetes is not controlled, the higher glucose level in the blood provides more fuel for the bacteria to "feed" on and hence to better multiply. The presence of a bacterial infection is stressful for your body, and in response the body produces "anti-stress" hormones to help fight the infection. These hormones (cortisol, adrenalin and noradrenalin, growth hormone, glucagon) increase your body's need for insulin, which if you are unable to make it yourself, leads to higher glucose levels. This becomes a vicious cycle as the higher the glucose, the better the bacteria grows and the infection worsens. Thus, it is very important to try to control blood glucose even better than usual when you have an infection, even if it means taking higher doses of insulin or tablets, or adding insulin to your usual regimen for a short time.

The kinds of infections that tend to occur in people with diabetes:

1. **Boils** are infections in the skin, often starting with a blocked hair follicle or duct for a skin oil gland. The body fights the bacteria with white blood cells and this "fight" will produce redness, inflammation, and pus under the skin. Pus is a combination of bacteria and the body's infection-fighting cells, as well as their breakdown products. Eventually, there is stretching and thinning of the skin over the area and the boil breaks open, releasing the pressure and pus. Once the boil opens, it is important that it empties completely so the bacteria causing the infection will not be left behind. The treatment of a boil is to try to bring the boil to a "head" where it is ready to break, which can be achieved by applying a warm compress for 5 to 10 minutes two to four times a day. A warm compress is easy to make using a clean facecloth, running it under water that is as hot as you can tolerate, squeezing out the extra water, and placing it over the site of the boil. Be careful not to get the water too hot—a burn won't help a boil! Sometimes big boils need to be opened surgically by a doctor.

2. **Yeast infections** occur where skin touches skin and is warm and moist, often in the inguinal areas (groin), the vaginal area, or under the breasts. In warm, moist areas, fungus that normally lives on the skin might begin to grow faster and establish an infection on the skin or the membranes inside the vagina. These infections are often associated with redness, raised areas, itchiness, and major discomfort. When they involve the vagina, they often result from yeast called candida albicans. Your doctor will give you antifungal ovules to insert and/or a cream. When the infection is on the skin's surface, an antifungal cream can be applied to the affected area.

3. **Balanitis** (infection under the foreskin of the penis) is often seen in men with diabetes. These infections can be fungal (similar to when a women gets candida vaginitis) or from bacteria. Either way, a visit to a doctor is needed to ensure prompt and appropriate treatment is started.

4. **Gum infections and cavities** are much more common in people with diabetes, especially when glucose levels are not well controlled. Visiting your dentist regularly for adequate cleaning, and to address any cavities or gum problems early, is a wise decision. As with virtually anything affecting diabetes, good glucose control limits problems in the mouth.

5. **Foot infections** are seen more frequently in the presence of diabetes.
   - **Athlete's foot,** a fungal infection of the skin of the foot, is the most common. This shows up as tiny blisters on the skin, cracking between the toes and, often, relative dryness of the feet and itchiness. At its worst, the entire sole of the

foot may be red, sore, itchy, and blistering. Although not a serious infection, athlete's foot should be treated, since the cracks that occur in the skin can provide an entry point for more serious bacterial infections. Often over-the-counter antifungal medications are available—your pharmacist can help you. The same antifungal creams that work for vaginitis or yeast infections in the inguinal fold areas will work for athlete's foot. It is wise to check with your doctor before using these medications in case the problem is actually something else.

• **Infection of blisters or cuts** can easily develop into a more serious infection such as cellulitis (infection of the tissue under the skin). Any foot infection can spread quickly in the presence of diabetes, especially if the blood glucose levels are elevated. This may then result in significant problems; thus a visit to your doctor or an emergency clinic is necessary as soon as infection is noticed. It is essential to check your feet for early signs of redness around small cuts or blisters. This is especially important if you have poor circulation or poor sensation in your feet, as your risk of gangrene and amputation is increased. More specific issues associated with foot care will be discussed in Chapter Nine.

## Ketoacidosis with or without Coma—A Rare Event, but Life Threatening

*Helene's story*

Helene is a young woman who has had type 1 diabetes for ten years. She has recently been in France, taking a final course before getting her degree. She was due to return home in three weeks, but she was running out of insulin. Instead of going to a pharmacy and/or doctor in France, she decided to take less and less insulin each day "to make it last." On the plane coming back to Canada, she started vomiting, had abdominal pain and could barely stand up. She was so sick she had to go directly to the hospital and was in the intensive care unit for three days with ketoacidosis.

We will follow Helene's progress throughout this chapter.

If you have type 1 diabetes, diabetic ketoacidosis (DKA) may be your introduction to the diagnosis. You become increasingly thirsty and hungry for glucose due to a severe lack of insulin (refer to Chapter Three). Glucose is unable to enter your cells so you make very little if any energy. The high glucose levels in the blood vessels flow through the kidney. This glucose is too much for the kidney to hang on to and the excess escapes into the urine. The urine glucose pulls out large amounts of water and other important salts or "electrolytes" that are essential in your blood. In particular, sodium chloride (NaCl or normal "salt") and potassium chloride (KCl) are lost to the urine, as well as phosphates. If you are vomiting, salts escape this way as well. Salt and water are important to keep blood pressure normal. If the body's stores of these salts are decreased too much, blood pressure will start to fall, making you dizzy when you stand up. The excess fluid loss also means your heart must beat faster to keep the few nutrients in your blood getting to the muscles, bones, liver, and brain.

If you experience such a severe insulin lack, you will feel exhausted, your heart will pound, you will have trouble standing up, and you will be extremely hungry and thirsty, especially for sweet things. There is not enough insulin to prevent the fat cells from releasing an alternate fuel or free fatty acids to the liver. If there is a significant lack of insulin, even these alternate fuels cannot be used, so energy production in the body is extremely low. As if that wasn't bad enough, without enough insulin your body transforms these free fatty acids broken down from fat cells into toxins in the form of acids called ketoacids. These acids, once they reach a very high level in your body, lower your blood pH to an "acid" level that blocks the work of essential enzymes and causes normal body functions to fail. If your body gets very dehydrated and the ketoacids build up too high, you might gradually lose consciousness or go into a coma. This process usually happens only when you have been really sick for hours or even days. In fact, ketoacidosis can lead to death if not recognized and treated, which is why people with type 1 diabetes died before insulin treatment was introduced.

Ketoacidosis must be treated in hospital with intravenous fluids, and might require a day or two in the intensive care unit. If caught early before becoming too severe, ketoacidosis may be treated in the emergency room.

Always, when anyone has had ketoacidosis, it is important to find out what caused it. Ketoacidosis can almost always be prevented if you know how to manage high glucose levels and sick days. The important thing to know is that, even if you are not eating much or even vomiting, you still require some insulin. One of the most common reasons for people to get ketoacidosis is that when they are unable to eat, they miss their insulin injections. Although the dose may be reduced by one half or one third, insulin should still be taken. (See details in the section on sick days later in this chapter.) Remember, if you do have ketoacidosis, the underlying cause must be treated as well as the ketoacidosis. For instance, if it was caused by appendicitis, a severe infection, or a heart attack, that must be treated also.

## What Will Cause Ketoacidosis?
- new-onset diabetes;
- acute illness (e.g., gastrointestinal flu);
- insulin omission/treatment errors;
- infection, (e.g., bladder, kidney, pneumonia, appendicitis);
- heart attack or stroke;
- inflammation of the pancreas (pancreatitis);
- street drugs or excessive alcohol;
- medications for other diseases (e.g., high-dose cortisone);
- insulin pump failure.

The symptoms of ketoacidosis are the same as those for high blood glucose, but as the ketoacidosis develops the symptoms become more exaggerated and others can appear.

Symptoms are:
- severe thirst;
- frequent urination;
- fatigue/weakness;
- nausea with or without vomiting;
- weight loss;
- abdominal pain;
- visual changes;
- leg cramps;
- somnolence—wanting to sleep all the time.

Ketoacidosis usually occurs only in people with severe insulin deficiency, that is, in people with type 1 diabetes. Occasionally it can occur in people with type 2 diabetes if they are so ill that they require much more insulin than they can produce, leaving them with a severe insulin deficiency. Whereas, a person with type 1 diabetes will always require insulin once he or she recovers, a few people with type 2 may be able to return to other forms of therapy once the underlying cause of the ketoacidosis is treated and resolved. The occurrence of ketoacidosis in a person with type 2 diabetes always suggests a certain lack of insulin, so once recovered, these people may do better and feel better with some insulin replacement if they were not already on insulin.

## Hyperglycemic Hyperosmolar Syndrome (HHS)

This condition comes on over days or even weeks and is life threatening. It is not uncommon, representing about 1 out of every 1,000 hospital admissions. Most people who develop HHS already have type 2 diabetes or glucose intolerance. More people die from HHS than from ketoacidosis because people who develop HHS are older and usually have other illnesses.

If you become very sick (for example, pneumonia, stroke, heart attack), you require much more insulin, as your stress hormones soar. Most people with type 2 diabetes have a reasonable amount of their own insulin, but in situations where they become very ill, they cannot possibly meet the increased insulin needs. Unlike ketoacidosis, where almost *no* insulin is available, in HHS, there is a significant lack of insulin, but just enough to prevent the fat cells from releasing the alternate fuel or free fatty acids to the liver. Thus the dangerous ketoacids do not accumulate. However, there is not enough insulin to allow the glucose to enter cells and the levels of glucose can go very high (above 30 mmol/L or 500 mg/dl). This causes you to become very dehydrated; your blood thickens and there is more chance of abnormal clotting of the blood. The extra water loss from your kidneys is often made worse by a decreased thirst (especially in older people) and therefore decreased fluid intake. This leads to a loss of blood volume that then can lead to the kidneys not working. If the glucose levels are very high, or dehydration is severe, you could go into a coma.

Your doctor must find and treat the underlying cause for your getting sick, which may be a heart attack, very severe infection (for example, kidney infection spreading to the blood), or stroke. The degree of severity—of the underlying disease that caused the increased insulin need—often relates to how well you will recover. Any person with very high blood glucose levels, who is not as alert as usual, should be taken to the hospital. The cause for the glucose going so high needs to be found and treated. In people with significant other illnesses and/or who are elderly, the mortality rate can be as high as 50 percent.

## The Lows: Hypoglycemia

Low blood glucose is called hypoglycemia, ("hypo" means below normal or low, "glycemia" means the level of glucose in the blood). Hypoglycemia occurs when there is too much insulin for the amount of glucose in the blood. People who do not have diabetes or who manage their diabetes with only diet and exercise, do not usually have hypoglycemia. Remember, the beta cells release a small amount of insulin throughout the day except when more is needed after a meal; therefore, a person normally would not have too much insulin.

### Reactive hypoglycemia

Some people, even those who do not have diabetes, can experience a hypoglycemic episode (low blood glucose) with symptoms. These people often have a prediabetes with a slow first phase insulin release, but intact second phase. After eating a large carbohydrate-containing meal, if first phase insulin is slow, the glucose level will go higher than usual. This results in a very large stimulus to release insulin but the insulin output may be too late for the peak glucose level, causing the blood glucose level to drop quickly to below normal levels.

Insulin, if taken in excess or not well-matched to food, can also cause hypoglycemia. When you take medication that stimulates your pancreas to release more insulin, it is possible that your blood glucose level will go too low. Medications that stimulate your pancreas to release more insulin are sulphonylureas and meglitinides.

Helene has recovered from her stay in hospital and returned to her active life in Montreal. She recently got a new job and finds that it takes her a long time to get there on the subway. One morning, she is in a hurry and leaves home without her usual purse. That morning, there was an accident on the subway and she realized that she had not eaten as much breakfast as usual and was feeling low. The longer she waited, the more shaky and uncomfortable she became. A young man sitting next to her realized she seemed distressed and asked if he could help. She explained that she had forgotten to bring candies with her and that her glucose level was going too low. Luckily he had a granola bar and a juice box in his backpack, which he gave her and she felt better. Soon after that, the subway started up again and she got to the office late, but OK. Next time, she will be sure to have her own glucose cache!

**What Will Put You at Risk for Hypoglycemia?**
- eating less than usual or later than usual;
- exercising more than usual without adjusting food intake or medication;
- more diabetes medication than usual;
- oral medications that stimulate insulin release too much;
- insulin doses that were excessive, badly timed, or the wrong kind;
- alcohol misuse (see later in the chapter);

- other diseases or changes in medications that might reduce insulin requirements (e.g., reduction of cortisone, decreasing kidney function).

## What Are the Symptoms and at What Glucose Levels Do They Occur?

Decreases in blood glucose trigger different responses as the level falls. The symptoms can be different in different people, and are often affected by how high or low your glucose usually is and the length of time that you have had diabetes. Commonly, the symptoms are as follows:

*Glucose Less Than or Equal to 3.8 mmol/L (68 mg/dl):*
Hormones called counter regulatory hormones are released to protect you by causing the liver to release stored glucose and interfering with the action of insulin. The counter regulatory hormones are:
- glucagon;
- epinephrine (adrenalin);
- cortisol.

There might not be symptoms at this stage, especially if the fall in glucose was slow.

*Glucose Less Than or Equal to 3.3 mmol/L (60 mg/dl):*
Start of the classic adrenergic symptoms (shakiness, sweating, palpitations, anxiety) related primarily to the release of the main counter regulatory hormone (epinephrine or adrenalin). These first symptoms are the same as when you have an "adrenalin rush" or are very frightened.

*Glucose Less Than or Equal to 2.8 mmol/L (50 mg/dl):*
Start of the symptoms due to the brain's inability to get enough glucose—these are called symptoms of neuroglycopenia ("neuro" means brain, "glyco" means glucose, "penia" means

deficiency or lack) and are a clear warning that the brain does not have enough glucose.

| Adrenergic Symptoms | Neuroglycopenic Symptoms |
|---|---|
| Initial symptoms usually | Usually occur later |
| • shaky<br>• sweating<br>• heart palpitations<br>• hunger<br>• nervous, anxious | • irritable<br>• headache<br>• blurred vision<br>• confused<br>• unresponsive |

## What Do I Do If My Blood Glucose Is Too Low?

It is very important that you know what to do and do it immediately when you feel the symptoms. Delay of treatment is risky as hypoglycemia develops quickly and you may become confused and unable to treat it. A hypoglycemic event is considered severe when you need help to treat it. You should make every effort to avoid getting to that low a value.

## How Do I Treat Hypoglycemia?

Mild hypoglycemia is very common and is not unexpected in any person who takes either insulin or an oral medication that stimulates the pancreas to release more insulin, such as a sulphonylurea or a meglitinide.

If possible, check the blood glucose to confirm a low blood glucose. If unable to check, it is always safer to treat as if your blood glucose is low.

1. If having symptoms and/or below 4 mmol/L (72 mg/dl) treat with 15 g of glucose:
   - 15 g of glucose in the form of tablets;
   - 3/4 cup (175 mL) regular soft drink or juice;
   - 1 cup (250 mL) milk;
   - 3 packages (15 mL) or 3 teaspoons of sugar;
   - 6 Lifesavers or other hard candies.

2. Check blood glucose again after 15 minutes; if still less than 4 mmol/L (72 mg/dl), treat again.

Once the blood glucose is above 4 mmol/L (72 mg/dl), it is important to keep it there. So if a meal is due, eat it. If your next meal is more than one hour away you should have a snack consisting of one serving of starch and one serving of protein, such as

- 6 soda crackers and 1 ounce (30 g) of cheese, or
- a slice of bread and 1 tbsp (15 mL) of peanut butter.

For anyone taking acarbose along with insulin, a sulphony-lurea, or a meglitinide, the absorption of many sugars and starches will be slowed from the intestine. If you are taking acarbose, low blood glucose must be treated with "glucose" as in glucose tablets or the sugar that is in milk (lactose).

People who manage their diabetes with meal planning and exercise, metformin, acarbose, or thiazolidinediones only rarely experience hypoglycemia unless these medications are combined with insulin or those medications that stimulate insulin release.

**What Is Severe Hypoglycemia and How Is It Treated?**
Severe hypoglycemia is defined as any hypoglycemic episode requiring the assistance of someone else to treat.

If you are conscious and able to swallow, you need 20 g of glucose instead of 15 g as stated above. You can find 20 g in the following:

- 1 cup (250 mL) of regular soft drink or juice;
- 4 sugar packets or 4 teaspoons (20 mL) of sugar;
- 8–10 Lifesavers or other hard candies.

Some people may have personality changes associated with severely low blood glucose and may refuse to take the needed glucose, or even become combative. In that case, or if you have become unresponsive, the person helping you should call an ambulance or 911. Whenever possible, someone who is either in your family or who is frequently with you, should know how to use a glucagon emergency kit.

The glucagon emergency kit (1 mg of glucagon) comes with a solution of sterile diluent in a syringe and a sterile vial containing powder. This is how they work.

- Remove the cap from the syringe and the cap from the vial. Inject the solution in the syringe into the vial.
- Gently shake the vial until the powder is well mixed with the solution.
- Draw the entire contents of the vial back into the syringe and inject it under the skin.

The injection is done in the same way that insulin would be given. Usually this injection will raise your blood glucose enough for you to wake up and take glucose by mouth. The effect of the glucagon is short lived, so it is very important that food and glucose be taken before the effect wears off. Many people will be nauseated or even vomit after the glucagon injection, and often will have a headache.

The use of a glucose gel or thick honey inserted between the cheek and the teeth may help, if glucagon is not available. Although some is absorbed by the mucous membrane lining of the mouth, it works best when swallowed. However, an unconscious person should not have anything, even liquids, put into the mouth, as the risk of choking is great.

Once the emergency team arrives or you are in the emergency room, glucose will usually be given intravenously.

## What Is Hypoglycemia Unawareness?

Hypoglycemia unawareness is when you no longer sense a low blood glucose until it is too late to react and treat it yourself. As previously discussed, the initial symptoms are mainly "adrenergic"—related to the fight or flight symptoms of adrenalin. You may develop a defect in the "adrenergic" hormonal response to hypoglycemia, particularly if you have had a recent severe hypoglycemic episode or recurrent hypoglycemia. This puts you at much greater risk of not being able to recognize hypoglycemia. Glucagon responses to hypoglycemia are blunted or lost after the first decade of type 1 diabetes, resulting in an increased difficulty in bringing the glucose back up. Once glucagon is gone, you are mainly dependent on adrenalin to raise your glucose. Symptoms can also be blunted when people take medication called beta-blockers used for treatment of high blood pressure or heart disease. A few people with diabetes have changes to the nerves that stimulate adrenalin and therefore lose the "adrenergic" symptoms. (This will be discussed in Chapter Nine.) If you do not feel adrenergic symptoms, the warning signs that the glucose level is falling are lost. The first sign of hypoglycemia will be when the glucose is so low that the brain doesn't work properly (neuroglycopenic symptoms). Sometimes the first symptom of hypoglycemia is confusion or coma. Obviously, this is a very dangerous situation.

Most people with hypoglycemic unawareness can regain the ability to sense the symptoms. This is done by carefully avoiding all hypoglycemic episodes, even mild ones, until the sense of low glucose is felt again. This may mean adjusting your target blood glucose level to slightly higher levels for a period of two to three months and relearning what signals your body sends out when your glucose is low.

### How Can I Prevent Hypoglycemia Recurring?

After the hypoglycemic episode is over, you should always try to figure out why it happened and if there is anything you can do to prevent another. Be sure that you:

- Know how to recognize hypoglycemia, checking glucose as often as necessary to be sure. Don't guess, check!
- Know how to avoid hypoglycemia. For instance, if you had been very active and this resulted in a low blood glucose, then next time you do the same activity you should either eat something first or, if on insulin, find out how to reduce the insulin to prevent the low.
- Teach family, friends, or co-workers how to help you if you have a severe hypoglycemic episode.
- Wear a Medic-Alert bracelet or equivalent to warn others if you need help.

## Adjustments: Taking Control of Your Diabetes by Self-Adjusting for Everyday Life's Events

*Yvonne's story*

Yvonne has been managing her diabetes for several years now. She takes insulin three times a day and her A1C is consistently about 7 percent. The only time she has difficulty in managing her diabetes is when the activities in her daily life change. The last time she went on holidays, she found her levels were fluctuating more than usual. On weekends, she hikes, but during the week, she has a desk job. How can Yvonne maintain her excellent blood glucose levels when her activities change so much? We will follow Yvonne through this section.

If you did exactly the same thing every day and ate the same food every day, you would find managing diabetes much easier. But this is simply not possible or even healthy. Diabetes should not run your life—you should be able to run your diabetes so that you can live the life you want to live and do the things you want to do. To do this you need to have a very good understanding of how your body works in relation to the insulin available. In this section, we will review some of the challenges that people run into in their daily lives that will affect their blood glucose control.

It is important however, that you discuss your challenges with your diabetes team. As every person with diabetes is different and requires different amounts of insulin or medications to accomplish the same result, there is no simple answer to the following challenges. You must take the suggestions and questions posed in this chapter to your doctor or health care team to determine the best action for your diabetes.

Whether or not you will make changes to your management plan will depend on how "intensively" you manage your diabetes. That is, the more involved you are in your daily management, counting carbohydrates, checking to adapt your dose of medications (whether it's by adjusting your oral medications or using insulin ratios or dose adjustment algorithms), the easier it will be for you to make adjustments. If you are taking insulin just once or twice a day or taking long-acting oral medications, there may not be many changes you can make except in your activities or meal plan.

Treatment of diabetes often needs adjustment.

• It might need to be adjusted day to day because, for most people, every day is not exactly the same. This could mean adjusting food or exercise for someone taking oral medications or the use of an insulin adjustment scale for someone on insulin. Perhaps on days when you work out you take less medication. This sort of adjustment would also be made if you had an illness that increased your blood glucose, raising your need for insulin, or if you were sick and unable to eat at all, perhaps lowering your insulin needs.

• It may need an adjustment of the overall basic or usual regimen because of changes in your routine. Daily schedules change with the season, school, or work timing. If your current medication, whether insulin or oral medications, is not meeting your needs and the result is consistently high or low glucose levels, you might need a change. Using "pattern management" you look for problems at specific times of the day and then change only the usual insulin affecting those times.

• It may need adjustment because of major changes in your daily routine, such as travel across several time zones, periods of fasting for medical tests, or a long hike. This will require you to know how your meals, exercise, and medications interact to allow problem solving.

### What Do I Need to Consider as I Adapt My Diabetes Management to Changes in My Day-to-Day Life?

*You should always check with your doctor before undertaking changes in your diabetes management.*

In order to make effective decisions about whether your oral medication or insulin dose needs adjustment, you will need to consider:

*Your present glucose level or glucose meter check result*
You cannot reliably assess your blood glucose level by how you feel. You should never make changes to your medication based on feelings; always use a meter to get an accurate glucose level.

*Your planned food intake*
For those on insulin, the amount of insulin that you require is planned in relation to the food that you are eating; the most important factor is the amount of carbohydrate in the meal. There are two ways to manage your carbohydrates:

**Consistent food intake**: You adjust your meal plans so that the amount of carbohydrates eaten at a given meal remains constant from day to day (for example, two portions of carbohydrates at lunch every day, although the actual food would change). This reduces the need for adjusting insulin or the medication dose, since the carbohydrates in the meal remain constant.

**Variable food intake**: You vary the insulin dose according to carbohydrate food intake; in other words, more insulin with more food.

**Qualitative**: You have a set insulin dose for your normal meal. You also have a predetermined scale telling you how much insulin to add or subtract from the usual for "a little more" or "a lot more" or "a little less" or "a lot less."

**Quantitative** (carbohydrate counting): As discussed in Chapter Four, you can learn from the dietitian the amount of carbohydrates in foods and actually calculate how many grams of carbohydrate you are eating. You and your doctor or diabetes educator would then determine how much insulin you need for every 10 or 15 g of carbohydrate. Then, at a meal when you decide how much carbohydrate you are going to eat, you can figure out how much insulin you will need to cover it.

*Your level of exercise or physical activity for the last few hours or the next few hours*

If you exercise more, you will require less insulin. You can either increase your food intake and/or reduce your insulin dosage. With experience, you can work out the number of units to be removed or added for a particular activity. You may need to adjust your dose before and after the exercise. Some health professionals suggest considering a change in the meal dose if the exercise is likely to occur within two hours of the meal, either before or after. This may vary depending on the type of insulin. If you use a pre-mixed insulin, you may need to decrease your whole dose in the morning or before supper by a few units. Some oral medications cause short-term insulin release and may need adjusting for exercise.

*Your level of stress*

If you are stressed, either psychologically or physically, insulin needs will usually increase.

**How Do I Adjust for Short-Term Events?**

Everyone will at some time have days that are unlike any other. Your insulin needs for those days will change. When you understand your needs, you can be proactive and keep your levels within target.

## Menstruation

The hormone changes that occur during the menstrual cycle can cause fluctuations in blood glucose levels. For some, there is a higher insulin need in the second half of the cycle, dipping quickly on day 1 or 2 of the period. Women who check often will notice different patterns on those days and can learn to make the right changes to insulin doses.

## Super-active days

You probably do more or less the same amount of activity on a typical day whether you are at work, school, or home. However, some days might have very different levels of activity. You could need a different insulin regimen or dose of oral medications for certain days, such as weekends or weekdays, workdays or days off. You should consider the following:

- Meal timing: will you sleep in, stay up very late?
- Level of activity: are you into sports or do you read all weekend?
- Alcohol intake.

Yvonne has been asked by friends to go cross-country skiing next Saturday. They are planning to take along a lunch and ski from 10 AM until about 4 PM. Yvonne is concerned about managing her blood glucose levels on a day with that much activity.

Activity usually results in lower blood glucose levels. The decrease in levels may occur at the time of the activity, or it may be delayed and occur up to about 12 hours or more after the activity. Yvonne will have to be prepared to treat hypoglycemia at any time during the day, but she can also make some changes to her insulin regimen to reduce the risk of hypoglycemia.

Yvonne should look at which of her insulin doses will be working best when she is skiing. She should reduce that insulin somewhat to account for her increased activity. There is no specific formula to figure out how much to reduce the insulin by; Yvonne will have to make an educated guess based on her previous experiences. She should also reduce the insulin that will be working during the night following this day of skiing. As she will probably have used up her stores of glucose in the liver and fatty tissues during the day, she is at risk of hypoglycemia until those stores have been replenished or for about 12 hours.

Yvonne decides to reduce her morning intermediate acting insulin by half, as it will be working during the late morning and early afternoon when she is likely to be skiing the hardest. She will take her meter with her, and carry it in an inside pocket next to her body where it will not get too cold. She knows that meters do not work when they are very cold. She is going to pack a high-carbohydrate, low–glycemic index lunch so that it will be absorbed throughout the afternoon. She will take along granola bars that will help her keep her glucose high for longer than candies if her level goes low.

She also decides to reduce her supper intermediate-acting insulin by one third and to have an extra snack before she goes to bed. As an extra precaution, she is going to set her alarm for 3 AM so she can do a quick check then just to be sure.

## If I Am on Tablets, Should I Adjust My Treatment for My Daily Activities?

Adjusting insulin for daily activities is commonly done, but adjustment of tablets is not as common and may or may not be recommended. Some doctors or health care teams are hesitant to suggest adjustment of tablets, but for some people it may be a good idea. Check with your doctor before making any changes.

> David, our accountant, and his buddies are planning a few days of hunting. This usually means a lot of extra walking, but also extra eating and more alcohol than usual. He wants to know what to do with his tablets for diabetes. Does he increase them or decrease them? What is the best thing to take into the woods with him to treat a low blood glucose?

When David goes to the woods with his buddies, many of the same tricks for treating hypoglycemia on a ski trail, which Yvonne used, would help on the hunting trail. Often the effect of exercise balances the effect of eating, but the added alcohol could increase David's risk for a low blood glucose on his usual tablets. David should be prepared by having appropriate, easily portable long-lasting glucose sources (for example, granola bars). Checking his blood glucose will help him decide whether to eat more or less. Keeping his glucose close to the normal range will give him the best energy to chase after the deer.

If David decided, as a New Year's resolution, to go to the gym regularly on Monday, Wednesday, and Friday during his lunch hour, he may need to reduce his glyburide to avoid having a hypoglycemic episode those afternoons and eating back all the calories he had "worked off." But, if his New Year's resolution fades and he goes off on a gourmet cruise vacation with his wife, he is likely not only to need his usual dose, but also more.

The more David understands about how his particular treatments work, the more likely it is that he will be able to make adjustments based on his activities and food. Because many of the pills for diabetes do not have an immediate effect on glucose by releasing insulin, adjusting these may not be helpful (for example, thiazolidinediones, metformin).

## What Does Alcohol Intake Do to My Diabetes?

Most people who have diabetes can include alcohol in their life if used in moderation. The recommended amounts are similar to amounts for those without diabetes. General recommendations are one to two drinks a day or fewer than 14 drinks a week for men and 9 drinks a week for women. Even in moderation, alcohol intake must be considered as a source of calories, and liquors, sweeter alcohols, or mixes should be considered as a part of the carbohydrate total for the meal.

For most people, small amounts of alcohol affect glucose control minimally. The most frequent concern is often delayed hypoglycemia. Alcohol is toxic to the liver and even in small amounts (one glass of wine), it can interfere with the ability of your liver to release glucose when your blood glucose is falling. Usually as your blood glucose starts to fall, your liver will sense it and release some glucose from its stores to protect you from hypoglycemia. If this process is blocked by the alcohol, the protective liver glucose output is blocked. This effect may be seen anytime in the night or even the next morning, so care needs to be taken that an overnight insulin dose is not too high. Often, having alcohol is associated with a social event or eating out, so the blood glucose may be higher as you go to bed. A natural response is for you to increase the overnight insulin to cover the higher bedtime glucose and skip your usual snack. This may result in your glucose being too low during the night or the next morning. It may be necessary to lower your bedtime dose and/or have a snack with protein before going to bed. Although more commonly seen in people with type 1 diabetes, lower nighttime or next-morning glucose levels after alcohol can be seen in any form of diabetes. If someone is lower in weight or not eating a lot of food, the effects of alcohol may be more pronounced the next day (for example, in small, older women who eat very little generally).

If you drink alcohol without eating, you run a higher risk of having a low glucose that evening. Because you are drinking, you may not recognize the symptoms of hypoglycemia and fail to treat it. The symptoms of being drunk and hypoglycemia are similar—slurry speech, blurry vision, confused, sleepy. If you have alcohol on your breath even from a small intake, others may assume that you are drunk and you may not get the help for hypoglycemia that you need.

Yvonne has been invited to a party for a friend. She knows there will be snack foods available at the party, and the evening will consist of dancing and drinking with all her friends. She plans to have a good dinner before she goes to the party, and then to pace her drinking. To do this she will alternate an alcoholic drink with a non-alcoholic drink. She will also be sure to eat some of the carbohydrate snacks with her alcoholic drinks. If she is dancing a lot, she will be sure to eat more to account for the increased exercise. With all the exercise of dancing plus the alcohol, she will likely reduce her night insulin slightly since the last time she was out like this, she had a low the next morning.

If you have spent an evening such as Yvonne has, you need to be aware of possible hypoglycemia the next morning.

> When David and his buddies went hunting, David checked his glucose one night after walking all day and eating a huge pasta and steak dinner. He was surprised to find it was almost normal and was pleased with himself for discussing adjustments of his pills with his doctor. That day he had taken only half of his usual dose of glyburide. The next morning, his glucose was even lower (he did have a few beers), so before he headed out on the trails, he made sure that he took even less of his glyburide (one quarter his usual dose), and went off with his friend Mike, both of them with their lunch and extra granola bars just in case.

## How Do I Manage the Patterns or Adjust the Basic or Usual Dose?

Pattern management simply means that you look at your blood glucose results over a period of time to see if there are any patterns in the results. That is, are your results always high at a specific time of day, or low at another time of day? To do pattern management properly you should try to be as consistent as possible with your activity and meals over a period of at least three days. Over that time you should check your blood glucose as often as possible but at least before each meal and at bedtime. If you can check after meals as well you will have even more information with which to work.

Then look at your results and see where you are out of range.

### Suzanne's story
Suzanne is a mother of two young children. She has had type 1 diabetes for about four years. Although she had very good

control when she was pregnant, she finds her A1C has been creeping up and now her blood glucose values are sometimes too high. Four days of checking show the following results.

| | Pre Bkft | Post Bkft | Pre Lunch | Post Lunch | Pre Supper | Post Supper | Bed-time | Comments |
|---|---|---|---|---|---|---|---|---|
| Mon | 6.8 mmol/L (122 mg/dl) | 9.4 (169) | 10.3 (185) | 12.5 (225) | 7.1 (128) | 9.8 (176) | | |
| Tues | 6.1 mmol/L (110 mg/dl) | 8.2 (147) | 11.4 (205) | 13.5 (243) | 7.9 (142) | | | |
| Wed | 6.4 mmol/L (115 mg/dl) | 7.6 (137) | 12.3 (275) | | | | | |
| Thurs | 5.7 mmol/L (103 mg/dl) | 8.2 (147) | 13.6 (245) | 15.4 (277) | 10.1 (182) | 15.3 (275) | | Pizza for supper |

Suzanne has decided with her health professionals to aim for between 4.5 and 7 mmol/L (80md/dl–126 mg/dl). What do you think of Suzanne's results? Is there any time where she is having a problem on a consistent basis?

- Her pre-breakfast results are less than 7 mmol/L.
- Her post-breakfast results are less than 10 mmol/L.
- Her pre-lunch results are all higher than 7 mmol/L.
- Her post-lunch result are all higher than 10 mmol/L.
- Two out of three pre-supper results are just a little high.
- One post-supper result is high and the comment tells us why.

The time she is having the most trouble seems to be before lunch. If those results were within target, her after-lunch results would probably improve and, possibly, her before-supper ones as well. Suzanne needs to determine what is affecting her before-lunch blood glucose results. Here are the questions she should ask herself:

Is it caused by food intake?

- Am I having an unnecessary snack in the morning?
- How long is the period between breakfast and lunch?
- Do I need a snack in that time?

Is this because the insulin I take is not working at the right time?

- What insulin am I on?
- What is the peak action time of that insulin?
- When am I giving it?

Scenario 1. Suzanne takes intermediate-acting and regular/soluble insulin in the morning and regular/soluble insulin at supper and intermediate insulin at bedtime. Her breakfast is at 6:30 AM, she takes her insulin at 6 AM, and she has a coffee and sandwich at 10 AM, and lunch at 12:30.

Her insulin appears to be working well for her breakfast meal as her after-breakfast levels are within target. She probably does need a snack between breakfast and lunch as there is a six-hour space there, but maybe she would be better with half a sandwich or something with fewer carbohydrates, such as a small yogurt and a fruit. If she increased the fiber and protein in her breakfast, she might not feel so hungry mid-morning and could manage with a smaller snack.

Increasing her regular/soluble insulin in the morning might improve her pre-lunch results but she would have to aware of the increased risk of hypoglycemia after breakfast.

Scenario 2. Suzanne takes a long-acting insulin at bedtime and a rapid-acting insulin before each meal. The timing of her meals is the same as in scenario 1.

Usually snacks are unnecessary when a person is taking rapid-acting insulin, so perhaps by not eating the morning snack, the pre-lunch blood glucose would improve. If, however, Suzanne is hungry mid-morning and wants a snack, there may be a lower-carbohydrate choice she could make that would result in better levels. Or, because she has six hours between breakfast and lunch, regular or soluble insulin at breakfast might be a better choice than the rapid-acting insulin.

As you can see, there is no one solution to Suzanne's problem; it will depend on many variables. All the variables should be considered and solutions tried until the target blood glucose levels are achieved. Health care teams are an invaluable resource to help you work through these issues. It will take some time to achieve target levels using pattern management but the end result will be worth it—better blood glucose results on a consistent day-to-day basis.

## If I Have Type 2 Diabetes and Am on Tablets or a Small Dose of Insulin, Is There Any Value to Pattern Management for Me?

Although day-to-day variations are less likely with type 2 diabetes than with type 1, there is often value in looking at overall patterns to help both you and your health care team manage your diabetes better.

*Trevor's story*
Scenario 1. Trevor has type 2 diabetes and is on a thiazolidinedione (TZD) and the lowest dose possible of repaglinide

before breakfast and supper. His last A1C was 7.3—not quite low enough. He doesn't like to check, but his doctor asks him to do it. They have worked out a compromise so that he checks his fasting glucose and the time that his glucose is likely to peak after each of his meals, but only once every 10 days (on the 10th, 20th, and 30th day of each month; February is the best month!).

He gets these results:

| | Pre Bkft | Post Bkft | Pre Lunch | Post Lunch | Pre Supper | Post Supper | Bed-time | Comments |
|---|---|---|---|---|---|---|---|---|
| March 10 | 6.8 mmol/L (122 mg/dl) | 9.4 (169) | | 7.9 (142) | | 10.3 (185) | | |
| March 20 | 6.1 mmol/L (110 mg/dl) | 8.2 (148) | | 6.9 (124) | | 15.4 (277) | | Pasta supper |
| March 30 | 6.4 mmol/L (115 mg/dl) | 7.6 (137) | | | | 11.7 (210) | | |

When his doctor sees these results, she first asks about Trevor's usual intake at supper. Trevor has been more careful than usual about the quality and quantity of his suppers, so he feels that is not causing the higher glucose levels. They decide that Trevor should increase his breakfast dose of repaglinide slightly and his supper dose a little more. If he has a pasta supper, he should take an extra pill of repaglinide. He will continue to try to walk his dog every day after supper and eat wisely.

Scenario 2. Trevor is taking a TZD (thiazolidinedione), metformin, and glimepiride, all at maximum doses. He has recently lost 20 pounds (9 kg). Despite all this, his A1C remains at 8.7 percent and his results are as follows:

| | Pre Bkft | Post Bkft | Pre Lunch | Post Lunch | Pre Supper | Post Supper | Bed-time | Comments |
|---|---|---|---|---|---|---|---|---|
| March 10 | 8.8 mmol/L (158 mg/dl) | 12.4 (223) | | 8.9 (160) | | 14.3 (257) | | |
| March 20 | 9.1 mmol/L (164 mg/dl) | 10.2 (183) | | 7.9 (142) | | 17.4 (313) | | Out for Chinese Food |
| March 30 | 9.4 mmol/L (169 mg/dl) | 11.6 (209) | | 11.3 (203) | | 14.7 (265) | | |

Trevor has almost as little energy as when he was initially diagnosed. His get up and go has got up and gone. When he looks over the results with his doctor, they both agree that he needs to take the next step and get the pen. He needs insulin. At the very least, he will start some insulin at bedtime or supper to lower the glucose in the morning. His doctor tells him how to gradually increase his dose every four days until his glucose is between 5 and 7 mmol/L (90–126 mg/dl) before breakfast. Once his glucose levels are in that target range his tablets may be more effective. If not, he will need additional insulin in the day. The first injection seemed tricky, but he learned quickly and finds it nowhere near as difficult as he imagined and ... it works. He doesn't have to look at those high glucose levels and feel dragged out anymore!

## Should I Adjust My Medication When Traveling?

Travel across time zones rarely requires adjustment to oral medications for diabetes, but usually requires adjustments to insulin doses. Going east, you will lose hours in the day, and going west your day has many more hours. An increase or decrease of two hours or less does not usually require an insulin adjustment. If the change is more than two hours, you will be more comfortable and have better blood glucose levels when an adjustment is made.

If you take tablets for diabetes, and are heading east (losing time), you may need to reduce your dose or even skip a dose of any medication that stimulates insulin release (sulphony-lureas and meglitinides). Insulin sensitizers would be taken at the usual time of day.

When you are on insulin, as with any change, the change you make should be individualized, because it will depend on what insulin you are taking and your usual food intake. Discuss your travel plans with your health care team to develop a plan that will work for you.

### Karen's story

Karen decides to go to England for a holiday. She lives in Toronto so there is a five-hour time difference. On the way to England she will lose five hours. Her flight leaves Toronto at 8 PM and arrives at 8:30 AM in London. She has to be at the airport at 6 PM. She is aware that she will be served supper on the plane at about 9:30 PM and a light breakfast at 7 AM London time.

Karen takes intermediate-acting and regular/soluble insulin in the morning, regular/soluble at supper, and intermediate-acting again at bedtime. On the day she travels she should take her usual morning insulin. She could hold off taking her supper regular/soluble insulin until before the supper is served on the plane, or she could decide to have supper in the airport and take the regular/soluble insulin prior to that meal. Her usual intermediate dose will have to be reduced to take into account the shortened night. This dose is usually taken twice a day and therefore is covering about 12 hours. As she will lose five hours, it would not be unreasonable to reduce this dose by half or one third and take it at the usual time. In the morning on the plane when breakfast is served she should take her usual morning dose as she is starting a new day. Of course, checking her blood glucose frequently on the trip will be important, and she should err on the side of slightly higher blood glucose levels than run the risk of lows.

When traveling west, the day becomes longer and may include extra meals. You should talk to your doctor or educator about how much extra insulin to take for an extra meal. It would usually be the regular/soluble insulin or rapid-acting insulin you would give for an extra dose as they both act for only a few hours. For those taking tablets, especially some of the shorter-acting sulphonylureas or meglitinides, an extra dose may be needed if there is an extra meal.

If you take insulin and are planning a long trip over several time zones, be sure to plan your insulin before you go to ensure you maintain reasonable glucose control throughout your trip. Be sure to take all your flight/travel information with you when you talk to your doctor or diabetes educator about adjusting for the trip. It may be helpful to create a timeline showing the time in the departing city, the period on the plane (or bus or train) and the corresponding time in the arrival city on a piece of paper side by side to help visualize the difference in time zones. You can pre-order diabetic meals on most flights.

Always bring your medications (for diabetes and any other conditions) and some food with you in your carry-on luggage! Never pack insulin in your regular suitcase to go into a hold of a plane, as it may freeze at high altitudes. Be sure to pack the following with you in your carry-on:

- source of fast-acting glucose;
- meter and supplies;
- insulin and syringes or pen;
- crackers and cheese, granola bars—an alternative to food; which you may or may not get on the plane these days.

Remember, your checked luggage may not arrive with you at your final destination!

X-ray machines at security do not affect meters. To explain the necessity of the syringes or pen needles, it is a good idea to have a note from your doctor explaining that you have diabetes and require insulin.

For travel by train or bus, the same suggestions apply, although access to food may be easier. When possible, take the opportunity to move or walk around. Any long-distance travel can lead to an increased risk of blood clots in the legs from spending long periods in the same position. People with diabetes are at slightly higher risk than others.

## What Do I Do if I Have to Fast for a Medical Test or Have Day surgery?

At some point everyone is asked to fast for a blood test. If you are asked to fast so that you must miss your evening snack or so that your breakfast is later than usual, you may need to adjust your insulin. This would be especially true if your usual fasting glucose level is on the low side. Ask your doctor or diabetes educator whether you should reduce your overnight intermediate- or long-acting insulin and by how much. You should also check your blood glucose prior to driving or going out, if you have skipped breakfast, just in case you are low. It is always safer to treat the low and rebook the test than to have an accident on the way.

Some people have to fast for more extensive tests, like X-rays or a colonoscopy or even day surgery. This will require some pre-planning to avoid problems whether you have type 1 or type 2 diabetes.

**If You Have Type 2 Diabetes ...** If you take tablets to stimulate the release of insulin (see Chapter Six), you may need to avoid taking them the day of the test (or even the day before if you have been giving a liquid diet for tests on your bowel). You may need to check your glucose much more than usual for a day or two around the exam or test. If you take insulin, this may be worrying as you will not be able to eat in the morning if your blood glucose is falling too low. Keep in mind the following if you have to fast:

- Be the first in line at the lab, or book the earliest appointment you can.
- If you do have a later appointment you may be wise to reduce your supper or evening intermediate-acting insulin the night before.
- Be sure to have a good snack just before you have to start fasting.
- Do not take your morning insulin until you know you can eat.
- Be sure to carry with you a source of fast-acting sugar so you can treat hypoglycemia, should it occur.
- If you are fasting for surgery be sure to tell the hospital staff exactly what medications you have taken and how much.
- Inform hospital staff if you feel your blood glucose is dropping.

Some diabetes medications, such as metformin, need to be stopped prior to X-ray tests that involve an injected dye. Metformin should be stopped 24 hours before the test and not restarted until 48 hours after the test.

**If You Have Type 1 Diabetes ...** the above information about taking insulin applies, but it is also very important that you help people understand that even if you do not eat, you will need insulin. Some centers have insulin infusion protocols to allow an intravenous supply of glucose consistently and a low dose of insulin intravenously until you are ready to eat again. For tests or day surgery when you may not be able to eat until near suppertime, this may be the best solution. If you will be able to eat within one to two hours of your usual morning insulin dose, you may be able to simply delay the dose. Your doctor or diabetes educator may suggest that you take a smaller dose of your morning intermediate-acting insulin and none of your regular or fast-acting insulin until you are ready to eat your breakfast/brunch. You may need to adjust the amount based on what you are likely to eat. If you do not do this routinely, you should develop a plan with your doctor.

**What To Do About Fasting for Religious Reasons?**
Many cultures and religions have special times of the year when fasting is important. *In all religions, the official teaching is that those whose health would be compromised by the fast need not do it.* However, many people feel a strong need to fast as part of their beliefs.

- Checking your blood glucose throughout the day will help you determine if your blood glucose is going too low or too high.

- If you have type 2 diabetes and are not on any medication, it is very unlikely there would be a problem with fasting.
- If you have type 2 and take oral medications, you may risk low blood glucose if you take the medication and do not eat. If you take repaglinide or nateglinide you should not take them if you are not going to eat a meal. Other medications should be either reduced or not taken depending on your blood glucose.
- If you have type 1 or type 2 diabetes and take insulin, you will need to consider decreasing the dose over the period you will not be eating. The basal (intermediate or long-acting) insulin may need to be reduced by one third to one half of usual. The bolus (rapid or short-acting) insulin should probably be skipped if the meal is to be skipped. Checking the blood glucose frequently will be your guide as to how much insulin to take and when.

## What Do I Do if I Am Sick?

Illness will usually result in higher blood glucose levels as the anti-stress hormones released cause increased amounts of glucose to be released from the liver and interfere with insulin's effect on the cells. However, in the case of some gastro intestinal illnesses with diarrhea and/or vomiting, the blood glucose may fall if you are unable to take in any food or drink.

Blood glucose checking is very important during an illness. If your blood glucose goes too high you can develop ketoacidosis, discussed earlier in this chapter. Ideally, while ill, glucose levels should stay between 6 and 10 mmol/L (110–180 mg/dl). If illness is managed properly with adequate fluids and insulin, you probably won't need to go to hospital, although sometimes it is necessary. Most importantly, with proper care and planning, you will avoid ketoacidosis.

## When You Are Ill—No MatterWhat Kind of Diabetes You Have

- **Check your blood glucose every two to four hours.** You need to know if your levels are going up or down so that you can treat the diabetes appropriately throughout the illness.
- **Check for ketones** (see page 87). If you do not have enough insulin, your cells will be unable to get the glucose and your body will start to burn fat in an effort to provide fuel to the cells. Particularly if you have type 1 diabetes, the severe insulin deficiency can lead to ketoacidosis.
- **Keep your fluid intake up.** Keep your fluids up and if you are not able to eat, try to take liquids with some sugar and some salt. Here are some examples of fluids with 15–20 g of glucose that are easy to sip on if you are ill:

  – 1 cup (250 mL) of juice (taken over an hour) (e.g., apple juice is easily tolerated);
  – 1/2 to 3/4 cup (125 mL to 175 mL) of regular soft drink (taken over an hour), (e.g., "flat" ginger-ale);
  – 1 cup (250 mL) of liquids with some sugar and salt, particularly if vomiting or diarrhea is a problem (e.g., soups, Pedialyte, Gatorade, salted rice water that can be made at home (2 cups [500 mL] of water boiled with 1/3 to 1/2 cup [75 mL to 125 mL] rice and 1 tsp [5 mL] salt for 20 minutes, then rice removed).

- **If blood glucose levels are high,** try to keep your fluids up with a combination of small amounts of the liquids above and water, broths, or clear soups. If your glucose is high or increasing, you likely need more insulin and may need to be seen in the emergency room.
- **Treat fever,** if needed with aspirin or acetaminophen. If it persists, be sure to consult a doctor.
- **Treat nausea/vomiting,** if needed, with medications taken either by mouth or by rectum. Check with your doctor if you can take dimenhydrinate, 50 mg (Gravol) by mouth or suppository (if vomiting). Sometimes taking dimenhydrinate 20 to 30 minutes before you try to eat or drink may help you keep liquids down.
- **If you take pills for diabetes, and you are unable to eat,** it may be safer to hold off taking the pills until you are able to keep food down.
- **If you take insulin for your diabetes, continue it.** Although it may not seem right to take insulin if you are vomiting it is very important to take at least half of it. Even though you may not be keeping much down in the way of food, your blood glucose levels are likely going up as a result of the stress hormones. You need your insulin. In fact, many people when they are sick might need more insulin than normal. Your basal insulin, the intermediate- or long-acting, will usually stay at the same dose, although initially you may decrease it by one third to one half of the normal dose until you know if your glucose is going up or down. Your bolus doses for meals can be decreased if you are eating less, but could equally well require an increase due to the stress of the illness.

Think in advance and, before you become ill, ask your doctor or diabetes educator about a sick day plan. Your plan should include instructions on how to adjust your medications if you are sick. This may include a plan for insulin adjustment or sliding scale or "corrective" doses of insulin to correct your glucose levels.

Put together a sick-day kit so that everything you will need will be available. Your kit should include:

1. thermometer;
2. check strips for your glucose meter;
3. lancets;
4. ketone strips for urine or blood ketone–checking meter;
5. dimenhydrinate (e.g., Gravol) pills or suppositories;
6. doctor's phone number;
7. instructions on how to adjust your insulin;
8. instructions on when to call the doctor.

Every two to three months, check over your sick-day kit to ensure that the strips are not outdated and that things have not been "borrowed" from it.

## Go to the Emergency Room or Contact Your Doctor If:

- Your blood glucose is consistently over 15 mmol/L for more than 12 hours.
- Ketones are in your urine for more than eight hours.
- You are vomiting and unable to keep anything down for six hours.
- You have fever and chills.
- You are ill and not improving.

## What About Over-the-Counter Medications? Can I Take Any?

There are many products at the pharmacy that you can buy to treat minor health problems. You should always ask the pharmacist if the product you are considering is appropriate for someone with diabetes. Here are a few things to keep in mind:

- Many products contain sugar or a sugar substance to make them taste good. Look at the label for words ending in "ose," such as dextrose, glucose, etc.
- Any product that says "syrup" will have sugar.
- Many products have a "sugar-free" option, such as Metamucil, Maalox, etc.
- Many products contain alcohol—be sure to read the labels.
- Many decongestants contain pseudo-ephedrine. This compound has adrenalin-like action, so it can increase slightly the need for insulin, which could cause a mild increase in your blood glucose. These are not recommended for people with diabetes.
- Be especially careful when buying products for foot care. Do not use anything that contains salicylic acid to peel away corns, calluses, or warts. These can easily peel away healthy tissue as well.

## What About "Natural" Health Products—Can I Use Them?

Natural products can be used with the advice of the pharmacist or doctor. Remember that even natural products will have side effects and can interact with your other medications. It is important that you tell your pharmacist and doctor about any natural products you are taking.

In this chapter we have explained some of the more severe and potentially life-threatening complications to be aware of so they can be avoided. We have also covered a few of the changes in daily life that are known to affect your diabetes management. Use your meter to discover how your glucose levels change as your activities change day to day. The more you know about *your* diabetes the better you will be able to manage your glucose levels.

# NINE

# Complications of Diabetes

As time goes by, and the disease is present for longer, concern arises in virtually everyone—what are my chances of getting complications? The complications of diabetes are often the most worrying part when learning about the disease. Although it takes time, most people do adjust to the day-to-day ups and downs that come with diabetes. However, in the back of the mind there remains a fear of future unknowns—the "complications." This may be worse if you have family members who have had vision loss, kidney failure, early heart attacks, strokes, or amputations due to their diabetes.

The good news is that we now know that these complications are not inevitable. The chances of the development and/or the progression of complications can be dramatically reduced by excellent control of blood glucose, blood pressure, and lipids. Remember, the complications of diabetes do not occur in people without diabetes. The microvascular complications of diabetes (eyes, kidneys, nerves) are known to be related to how high and how long glucose levels have been elevated. The degree of glucose control is also related to the development of macrovascular complications such as heart attacks and strokes.

### James's story

At 62, James has known that he has diabetes since he was 55. Initially, the tablets worked, but for the last year, he has needed insulin. He always found diabetes hard to deal with—this business of avoiding eating certain foods and the extra effort involved. He has downplayed the diabetes and tries to ignore it. But lately, it's harder to ignore as he notices that his feet seem to burn at night and he has to get out of bed and walk on the cold floor for it to stop. But even more annoying is the vague sense of pressure in his chest when he's walking up the hill on the 17th hole of the golf course. He seems to tire so quickly these days.

### Marian's story

At 33, Marian is an energetic young teacher, enjoying her class and her friends. She has been married for four years and she and her husband are considering starting a family. Because she has had diabetes for 22 years, she went to the doctor for a checkup before getting pregnant. The doctor asked her to see an ophthalmologist before making the decision to get pregnant. Her ophthalmologist looks concerned. Marian has changes in her eyes from diabetes that need to be treated before she gets pregnant.

One of the major advances in prevention has been the recognition that routine screening for any early evidence of complications is very important. Most complications start without any symptoms but can be treated if they are caught early enough. Early treatment of complications may prevent progression or even reverse some damage. Read on to find out more about screening tests you should have regularly.

Some people with type 2 diabetes may already have diabetic complications at the time they are diagnosed. This is because they may have had high glucose levels for up to about seven years before they are diagnosed. In fact, the symptoms associated with the complication may be the reason the diagnosis of diabetes is made.

Even if you have complications, optimal glucose control can decrease their severity. Periods of exceptionally good glucose control appear to have prolonged effects that can last years, (a metabolic memory) providing further protection against complications, even if glucose levels go a bit higher from time to time. This is a very good reason to aim for the best possible glucose values early on in your diabetes, since every year of great glucose control counts in reducing the risk of development or progression of complications!

## Macrovascular Complications—Large Vessel Disease

The large-vessel complications result from a condition called **atherosclerosis** ("athero" means vessel, "sclerosis" means blocked or closed due to scarring). Atherosclerosis is a ticking bomb that starts before the diagnosis of diabetes. The life expectancy for people with diabetes is shortened by about 10 years, mainly due to vascular events such as a heart attack or stroke. Atherosclerosis applies to blockages of the blood vessels:

*In the heart—cardiovascular diseases:*
- angina (pain in the heart muscle from lack of blood flow);
- heart attack or myocardial infarction (MI), which means an area of the muscle of the heart loses its blood supply so that heart muscle cells die.

*In the brain—cerebrovascular diseases:*

- a transient ischemic attack (TIA)—area with decreased blood flow for a short-time causing temporary changes in sensation or brain function;
- a stroke or cerebrovascular accident (CVA)—where an area of brain cells dies from lack of blood flow.

*In the legs—peripheral vascular diseases:*

- "claudication" or pain during walking that clears during rest, due to inadequate blood flow;
- gangrene when the blood supply is completely blocked so the cells die.

Macrovascular complications pose the biggest threat in both types 1 and 2 diabetes, accounting for the majority of deaths. More than 75 percent of people with diabetes will die from a vascular event. In the years prior to the onset of diabetes, many people have had either impaired fasting blood glucose or impaired glucose tolerance (see Chapter Three). The presence of a cluster of abnormalities that include mild elevations of blood glucose with a bigger waist (high abdominal fat), low protective blood lipids and high triglycerides, higher blood pressure as well as some other abnormalities (metabolic syndrome, see Chapter Three) have been associated with higher atherosclerotic risks even before diabetes is diagnosed. The bottom line is that it is never too early to adjust your lifestyle and consider preventive therapies when blood glucose is abnormal.

### Am I More at Risk of Having a Heart Attack?

In large studies, the presence of diabetes doubled the risk of cardiovascular disease in men. Women with diabetes have a marked increase risk of cardiovascular disease compared with women of the same age without diabetes. A woman with diabetes has the same degree of risk of having a vascular event as a man with diabetes—she loses her gender advantage. In the presence of type 2 diabetes, men aged 45 and older and women aged 50 and older are considered at high risk for having or developing cardiovascular disease. In type 1 diabetes, individuals aged 30 and older are considered high risk if they have had diabetes longer than 15 years. In addition, if you have diabetes and any other risk factor (advancing age, hypertension, sedentary lifestyle, abnormal obesity, smoking, high LDL [bad fats]), sedentary lifestyle, abnormal obesity, your risk of cardiovascular disease increases more than it would in someone without diabetes. Not only are the chances of heart attacks increased, but also the symptoms of chest pain are decreased, making you less aware of something being wrong with your heart. This puts you at an even greater risk of having something wrong with your heart and not realizing it. Early diagnosis and either angioplasty (blood vessels are opened by a balloon inserted in a narrowed coronary [heart] vessel) or coronary artery bypass surgery can be done and will help preserve a healthy heart muscle.

The important thing is to recognize a problem with the circulation to the heart before a blood vessel blocks and heart muscle actually dies (a myocardial infarction). Unfortunately, not only is there a greater chance that you will have a heart attack if diabetes exists, but also the chances of complications occurring in relation to the heart attack are higher. This means there may be more chance of heart failure and the requirement for more medication. The good news is that the risk of having a heart attack in the North American population has decreased during the last 50 years for people with and without diabetes. The bad news is that people with diabetes still have a two- to three-fold greater risk.

James goes to see his doctor who insists that James undergo a stress electrocardiogram and a special ultrasound scan of his heart. Based on these tests, the doctor diagnoses angina and hypertension. This accounts for the pressure James feels in his chest when climbing the hills. The doctor encourages James to make some changes to his lifestyle and start to take his diabetes seriously. She gives James a prescription for an antihypertensive medication, which will also lower the risk of angina, and some nitroglycerin to take when he senses the pressure in his chest. She reminds James to take the lipid-lowering pill that he stopped and to start back on the low-dose aspirin that he rarely takes. She refers him back to the diabetes education center—for some help in getting back on track with the day-to-day management of his diabetes—and to a cardiologist.

---

### How Can I Best Prevent Troubles? Investigate Symptoms Early, Don't Procrastinate!

Early indications of heart disease can be easy to ignore or miss altogether. They may include:

- Significant increase in fatigue or not being able to do activities without being short of breath;
- Chest discomfort that can feel like indigestion;
- An ache in the neck or arm when active that can indicate heart trouble but is put off as being muscular.

It is important not to be neurotic, but at the same time, not to ignore early symptoms. Early symptoms may indicate that the heart has inadequate blood supply when demand increases. Talk to your doctor about any symptoms you have.

---

### What Are My Chances of Having a Stroke?

In the United States, of those who have been discharged from hospital with a stroke, about 20 percent have diabetes. Looking at this from the other direction, of all hospital discharges of people with diabetes, 11 percent of them were due to strokes. The chance of having a stroke (or any other "vascular" event affecting the brain) is increased by two to three times in people with diabetes, even when all the other factors that would increase the risk are taken into account. Again, the presence of any of the other risk factors such as high blood pressure and the degree that they are controlled play a bigger role in people with diabetes than in those who don't have it.

### How Can I Avoid the Possibility of an Amputation?

Foot problems are an important cause of concern for people with diabetes. This is often because nerve changes are common (more than half of people aged over 60 with diabetes will have this problem). Changes in large and small blood vessels that supply blood to the legs are also more common if you have diabetes; The length of time that you have diabetes, how well it was controlled over those years; and whether you smoke or have smoked, have hypertension; or have abnormal lipids will all affect your risk of this complication. If you have had diabetes fewer than five years, the risk of peripheral vascular disease is 1.4 times higher than those without diabetes; after 25 years, the risk is 4 to 5 times those who have similar other risk factors but no diabetes.

The best protection for your feet, above and beyond the overall risk factor control discussed below, is to exercise, since that helps promote normal blood flow, and to check your feet daily, especially if you have nerve or blood vessel disease in your legs.

### What Causes the Blockage?

Large blood vessel disease (macrovascular) is due to changes in the walls of the arteries. These changes are due to a combination of the build-up of cholesterol and cells caused by inflammation, and high levels of blood fats. Why does it occur more frequently in diabetes?

- Insulin does many things apart from helping glucose get into cells. It helps certain enzymes in your blood deliver fat to your cells. When there is not enough insulin, cholesterol and triglycerides can build up in the blood as glucose does. People who have high levels of bad cholesterol (Low Density Lipoprotein or LDL) or low levels of good cholesterol (High Density Lipoprotein or HDL) are at higher risk of macrovascular disease. Genetics also plays a role—some people have a genetic predisposition to abnormal lipid levels. The more appropriate the levels of insulin for glucose control, the more likely fat delivery to the cells is normal and the less it will build up in the blood. An active lifestyle, eating a diet relatively low in saturated and trans fats, and not smoking will all help improve the blood fats.
- Damage may also be caused to the walls of the blood vessels by inflammation or by some local tissue chemicals that may result from high glucose levels. The damaged blood vessel walls may not respond to changing needs of blood flow as easily. See Chapter Three for more on this. Inflammatory change can be assessed indirectly by measuring the C-reactive protein (or highly sensitive CRP). This goes up when there is inflammation occurring at the level of the vessel wall.
- Lack of insulin, high blood glucose, and some genetic influences also increase the chance of clots forming. Since the final process that blocks an artery is often a clot (or "thrombus"), this clearly is important. The first stage of

a clot forming is when tiny partial cells in the blood called platelets start sticking to each other, releasing substances that encourage further clotting.

The more normal the glucose, the better the blood fats, the less inflammation present, and the lower the thrombotic tendencies, the lower the overall risk of macrovascular disease will be. The combination of these risks is not insignificant and each is worth fighting to decrease. We know that many of these changes actually start *before* diabetes is diagnosed; therefore, treatment and prevention of vascular disease is extremely important. A recent report from a large trial (the Diabetes Control and Complications Trial—EDIC) of optimal versus standard levels of glucose control in people with type 1 diabetes, has shown that good glucose control can reduce the number of heart attacks and strokes. The protective effect of good glucose control had already been an accepted concept from studies done earlier in people with type 2 diabetes. In both type 1 and type 2 the people with the most elements of the metabolic syndrome are likely to have the highest risk of cardiovascular disease (See Chapter One).

## What Does All This Mean to You?

### Control Glucose

The better your insulin fits your glucose needs, the better your levels of blood glucose, cholesterol, and triglycerides will be. A recent long-term study in people with type 1 diabetes showed that control of blood glucose was the most effective preventive measure, even more effective than cholesterol-lowering medication, to avoid long-term complications. Also, good blood glucose control usually means that you will have a reduced tendency to make clots or have abnormal lipids.

Although good glucose control helps prevent problems, if efforts to reach better control lead to recurrent or severe hypoglycemia, the risks for worsening cardiovascular outcomes can increase. Caution is essential to avoid hypoglycemia.

**Control Blood Pressure**

People with diabetes, especially type 2, are at higher risk of having high blood pressure. Up to 70 percent of people with type 2 diabetes are hypertensive. Studies have shown that the better the control of blood pressure, the lower the risk of heart attacks and stokes. If the pressure in the blood vessel is increased, each time the heart beats, there is potential for damage to the inside of the blood vessel, increasing the chances of worsening atherosclerosis. Think of the blood coming down the blood vessel like waves that hit land and over time, eventually change the shape of the land.

Initial treatment for elevated blood pressure involves a healthy meal plan, often with lowered salt intake, and regular physical activity. Usually people with diabetes require medication to improve blood pressure.

Blood pressure treatment can require more than one kind of medication. The major types of medications used are:

- Angiotensin-converting enzyme inhibitors (ACE inhibitors) lower angiotensin, which is a substance that stimulates contraction in the small arteries of the body. It is particularly helpful in the kidneys where, by relaxing the small vessels, it decreases the pressure in the kidney filters, resulting in less loss of protein. As well, it has been shown to protect the heart. Most people tolerate this medication very well. About 5 percent of people may get a dry irritating cough with this medication. This will not make you sick but it can become difficult to live with and may make it impossible to take this medication.

- Angiotensin receptor blockers (ARBs) act to block the way angiotensin causes contraction of the blood vessels, similar to how the ACE inhibitors work. Thus, they also protect the kidney and the heart. They do not produce a cough, so in some people they are better tolerated.
- Water pills or diuretics encourage excess salt (sodium) to be removed from the body, which often helps lower the systolic (top number) pressure.
- Calcium-channel blockers decrease the ability of blood vessels to contract, often particularly helping the systolic blood pressure.
- Beta-blockers block the blood vessel contraction effect of adrenalin, resulting in reduced ability of the blood vessel to contract. They can interfere with the normal adrenalin response to a low blood glucose and can worsen asthma, so they cannot always be used.
- Less frequently used medications act in the brain and where the nerves reach the blood vessels, decreasing vessel contractions. Other medications can have direct effects on blood vessels to relax them, rather than blocking their contractions.

There may be other rare side effects to these medications than are mentioned here. Your doctor will work with you to find the best combination of medications to control your blood pressure with the minimum of side effects.

### Don't Smoke

Smoking in itself has no effect on blood glucose levels; however, it is certainly not recommended for people with diabetes. As in all people, smoking constricts the blood vessels, causes the platelets to become sticky, decreases oxygen available for tissues and damages the lungs. For people with diabetes who already have an increased risk of heart disease, smoking could be compared to playing with fire. The bottom line is *do not smoke!*

## Control Lipids

It has been shown that even small elevations of bad cholesterol (LDL) or decreases of good cholesterol (HDL) should be treated. The first step is healthy eating and increased physical activity. Major changes in the type of fat and overall fat intake must be made, and activity, to be effective for blood fat improvement, must be almost daily and significant. However, as only about one third of cholesterol actually comes from food and the rest comes from your liver processing the fat sent from the fat cells, it is not easy to achieve normal cholesterol or triglyceride levels with decreased fat intake and activity. Stopping smoking will result in higher HDL levels, increasing your protection from vascular diseases—another excellent reason to be a non-smoker.

People who are not able to achieve target blood lipid levels need to take medication.

- Statins block the body's formation of fats in the liver. These are used if LDL is too high.
- Fibrates are used if the HDL is low, or triglycerides are very high.
- Niacin may help increase HDL, but may interfere slightly with insulin release, so sometimes can cause increases in glucose. This could require changes in glucose medications.
- Ezetimibe interferes with the re-absorption of cholesterol in the gut, so improves the action of statins or can be used by itself to lower LDL cholesterol.

## Eat a Heart-Healthy Diet

Most diets recommended for diabetes are inherently heart healthy. Here are a few specifics to make your diet more heart healthy.

- Follow a diet that is lower in saturated fats, trans fats, and cholesterol than before diagnosis. This includes animal fats and hydrogenated fats. Substituting fish for meat will help reduce the saturated fats and increase the omega-3 fatty acids, which are felt to be protective.
- Eat more fiber—more than 25 grams a day. Fiber is found in whole grains, fruits, and vegetables.
- Eat lots of fruits and vegetables—up to 5 to 10 servings a day.
- Add some nuts and seeds to your meals—about 2 tablespoons five times a week.
- Use low-fat dairy products.
- Limit salt use.
- Limit alcohol, especially if blood pressure is high.

For more information about combining a heart-healthy way of eating with your diabetes meal plan, speak to your registered dietitian.

## Become Physically Active

Physical activity helps on every front in decreasing cardiovascular risk: decreases blood glucose, blood pressure, LDL, insulin needs, and increases HDL, etc. Refer to Chapter Five for more suggestions for physical activity.

## Take Acetylsalicylic Acid (ASA)

Acetylsalyclic Acid acts by making the platelets less sticky, so they do not clump together. The clumped platelets produce other substances that may promote the formation of clots and hence blockage in the vessels. It is recommended that most people with diabetes and cardiovascular disease take a small dose of aspirin (80 to 325 mg/day) to avoid small clots becoming big ones. Of course, if you are allergic to aspirin, you cannot take it. An alternative product exists (clopidogrel) for those people who need antiplatelet action but are allergic to aspirin. In certain situations, it is used by preference.

> James returns to his doctor for a follow-up. He has restarted his meal plan and taken the blood pressure medication. He has not managed to make it to the cardiologist yet. It seems the appointment was the same day as a golf game and he didn't go. The doctor strongly encourages James to make the cardiology appointment a priority. She reminds him that his stress electrocardiogram (ECG) was abnormal and that, unfortunately, half the people who have their first heart attack never make it to the hospital. The doctor remakes the cardiology appointment, since James really needs an angiogram to evaluate the vessels to his heart. He may need an angioplasty or a cardiac bypass operation. She reminds him to use the nitro spray if he gets "indigestion" since it actually increases the flow of blood to the heart and improves the circulation. It's not a "pain" pill but treats the immediate problem. She suggests that James "listen to his body," reducing his activities if he has any discomfort until he is sure that his heart is fine. If he's in doubt about chest discomfort, he should go to the emergency room.

**Reduce Risk for Blood-Vessel Disease**

- Control glucose effectively.
- Control high blood pressure optimally.
- Don't smoke.
- Control blood fats with medications as needed.
- Eat a heart-healthy diet.
- Exercise regularly.
- Discuss low-dose acetylsalicylic acid (ASA) with your doctor.
- Attain or maintain a healthy weight.

## Microvascular Complications— Small-Vessel Disease

What about microvascular or small-vessel diseases? The diagnostic glucose levels for diabetes are based on the levels where complications, particularly in the eyes, begin to develop. People without diabetes can have heart attacks, strokes, even gangrene and amputations, but the complications related to small-blood vessel disease occur only in people who have diabetes. They are called "micro" vascular because they occur in the very small blood vessels (arterioles, capillaries, and venules) where the transfer of nutrients (oxygen, glucose, and amino acids) occurs in the cells.

Some of these abnormalities (retinal changes, nerve damage, and, more rarely, kidney damage) may be present at diagnosis in people with type 2 diabetes. This is because they have often had diabetes on average seven years prior to it being diagnosed, as discussed previously.

In people with type 1 diabetes, there is the potential for these complications to start at an early age. The changes leading to complications tend to begin after puberty and often require at least 10 to 15 years to develop, so that they may be seen as early as age 20 in those with very early onset diabetes. These days, with improvements in insulin and its delivery systems as well as a better understanding of the disease, many people with type 1 diabetes are free of complications despite having had the disease for 30, 40, 50 and even 60 years. To achieve this, however, requires a major commitment to diabetes control that must never be relaxed.

### What Causes the Microvascular Complications?

Excess glucose in the blood will attach to various other molecules in the blood, causing them to be "glycated"—to have extra glucose attached. These molecules are involved in many processes within the body, both within the blood vessels and in the surrounding tissues. The glycated molecules behave differently than the original molecule. An example of this is the glycated hemoglobin molecule, called the "A1C" molecule, which is used as a measure of glucose control. When glycated hemoglobin molecules reach the tissues, they do not release oxygen to the tissues as easily as the non-glycated hemoglobin molecule. This means that, at a microscopic level, the higher the blood glucose, the higher the percentage of glycated hemoglobin, and the less oxygen the tissues will get. If this goes on long enough, areas in the tissues either won't work well or they die (micro-infarcts).

Proteins other than hemoglobin can also have extra glucose attached. As a group these are called **advanced glycated end products**, or AGEs for short. Over time and with high glucose, these build up and interfere with or block normal functions. Efforts to find medications that interfere with the formation of AGEs are ongoing, but, so far, the best method known is to keep glucose levels as close to normal as possible.

Overall there tends to be a breakdown of the functioning and repair processes that keep our body working effectively if glucose is elevated or insulin is deficient or both. The effect is to speed up the aging process of various parts of the body.

# What Are the Microvascular Complications?

## 1. Retinopathy

"Retina" is the back of the eye where nerve cells "sense light" allowing us to see; "pathy" means disease or morbid condition. Retinopathy is a major cause of disability in patients with diabetes. Loss of vision, whether in a limited way or as severe as blindness, is no small matter. In the western world, diabetes is the most common cause of adult blindness. Most people with diabetes have no symptoms until the very late stages (by which time it may be too late for effective treatment). This is why it is so important to have regular eye examinations by a qualified specialist, such as an ophthalmologist or optometrist trained to examine the back of the eye after the pupil has been dilated. Treatment of eye disease can be effective, as long as it occurs early enough in the process to stop progression of the problem. Without an eye exam, you might not know you have a problem until it is too late.

Studies in both type 1 and type 2 diabetes indicate that the development of retinopathy and its progression are clearly related to elevated blood glucose levels and the length of time they have been elevated. In those who are well controlled, it may take 15 to 20 years to develop any changes at all. With good glucose control, any further changes seen in the eye may progress very slowly. However, in the presence of markedly elevated glucose levels, changes can occur very quickly. Overall, for each 1 percent decrease in A1C, there can be a 37 percent drop in diabetic eye disease.

Although there is no doubt that good glucose control will increase the long-term chances of good vision, sudden improvements from moderately poor to very good control (such as in early pregnancy or after a decision to dramatically control glucose levels), can cause retinopathy to progress more rapidly for a short time. This is why women considering pregnancy benefit from improving their glucose control prior to getting pregnant. It is also wise to improve from very poor control to very good control in steps, gradually bringing down the glucose levels and A1C over a number of months, rather than within one to two months.

**What Happens with Diabetes That Causes Visual Changes?**
The back of the eye where specialized cells that sense light are placed (the retina) is a very busy place. Changes in the hormone balance and/or blood flow can interfere with how these important cells work. There are various terms used to describe the degree of change that the eye doctor can see in your eye.

*Background retinopathy*
At first, the changes in the eye result in no change to your vision. The tiny vessels that feed the retina become weakened and start to leak, resulting in spots called exudates that may be protein or lipids (blood fats). Small bumps called microaneurysms may develop on the vessels. These are visible only to the doctor who looks in your eye with an ophthalmoscope.

*Pre-proliferative retinopathy*
This next stage is a result of deteriorating blood flow to the retina:

- Some cells will die because they do not have enough oxygen.
- The cells that are sick or dying will look white (cotton-wool spots).

- The sick cells will release various chemicals that stimulate other cells to grow to make new blood vessels.

There can be multiple hemorrhages and beading on the vessels as well as branching out of vessels in the retina. Tiny amounts of bleeding can occur, usually within the retinal layer. Evidence of new vessels forming within the layers of the retina can be seen (IRMA or intra-retinal micro-aneurysms). These changes indicate a significant potential for visual loss, although you may *still not notice any real change of vision*. At this point, it is essential that you be evaluated by a qualified retinal specialist. Prompt treatment with laser photocoagulation may be necessary to save your vision. When this stage is reached, regular follow-up appointments are vital.

*Proliferative retinopathy*
This stage is characterized by the growth of the new vessels, some of which grow into the vitreous area (gel-like substance in front of the retina). Vessels in the vitreous are unsupported and weak. They can bleed very easily; for instance, if there was a sudden change in blood pressure or a sudden movement. When there is a bleed into the vitreous area, your vision is impaired because you cannot see through blood. Usually the blood will clear up gradually on its own. Sometimes a scar forms (similar to what happens when you scrape your knee and the scar puckers up) pulling the retina away from its connection with the brain so no light can register in the area. This would produce a blind spot in your vision. An operation to replace the blood in the vitreous with clear fluid and/or to break any scars that may be pulling the back of the eye away may improve vision even after a retinal bleed occurs. This operation is called a vitrectomy.

Marian has found out from her ophthalmologist that she has proliferative retinopathy; there are some new blood vessels developing in the back of her eyes. The ophthalmologist tells her she that she needs laser treatment to prevent those new vessels from bleeding before she gets pregnant. Marian decides to go ahead with the treatments and to wait another six months before getting pregnant. She progressively brings her A1C down and makes sure her eyes are "quiescent"—that her dangerous new vessel changes have resolved. She dearly wants to have a child but she also wants to protect her vision and realizes that she needs to be well prepared for the pregnancy.

## Macular edema

In many people with type 2 diabetes, retinopathy may not be such a problem, but there may be swelling of the retina in the macula. The macula is the most important area in the center of the retina that allows us to see color and details. If swelling occurs in this area, these macular cells can degenerate and central vision deteriorates or is lost. These changes are called "macular degeneration."

## How Is Retinopathy Treated?

The most effective treatment to prevent progression of retinopathy is glucose control. The other factors for prevention of microvascular complications are also important, such as blood pressure control, no-smoking, and blood lipid normalization.

When there are new vessels and they are in the pre-proliferative stage, treatment by laser photocoagulation has been shown to save vision. It may seem counterintuitive to "burn" tiny holes in the retina to help vision but it does work. The tiny burn holes are generally done in patterns around the outside of the eye. This decreases the overall need for blood to the eye, allowing better blood flow to the areas in the center of the retina that sense detail and color. The resulting decrease in requirements for nourishment to the retina also seems to "quiet" growth factors. Avoiding strenuous exercise when you have active eye disease and particularly after laser treatment is important.

People with diabetes also have a tendency to develop cataracts more often and a bit earlier. Cataracts are simply the natural thickening and clouding of the lens of the eye. The lens in your eye normally focuses the light on the retina. When the lens is thickened, you cannot see well. The removal and replacement of cataracts with an artificial lens is done about as easily in people with well-controlled diabetes as with those without diabetes. If diabetes is poorly controlled, risk of infection of the eye area is increased.

## 2. Nephropathy

"Nephro" means kidney, "pathy" means disease or morbid condition. The kidney is your body's filter or blood cleaning system, controlling the nutrients you keep, the wastes that you excrete, and the levels of various salts in the blood that are essential for your body to function. The filtering is done from the nephrons into the tubules. The nephrons are clumps of blood vessels with very thin walls combined with tubules, which also have very thin walls. Materials that we need and those we want to get rid of flow back and forth across these walls. Molecules flow from the blood into the tubule. What the body wants to preserve will be pulled back into the blood. What it wants to excrete will stay in the tubule. Eventually, the tubule empties its contents into the ureter (the thin tube that connects the kidney to the bladder) and it leaves as urine. One of the important molecules that moves across the membrane is glucose, but it is an important fuel for the body so, usually, it is all pulled back to the blood and there is no glucose in the urine.

This filter system usually has very small holes, so that larger molecules like proteins that must stay in the blood, do stay. If there is a gradual glycosylation (attachment of sugars) in the area where the filtering occurs (called the mesangium), the filter process becomes leaky to proteins. Proteins need to stay in the blood to pull back some of the other substances. If proteins are lost, the whole process becomes less effective and some of the body's waste products will not be excreted. As well, the small blood vessels can begin to be blocked in the tiny capsule where the filtering occurs and pressure in the small blood vessels may increase, changing the way the blood is filtered. These changes lead to the release of substances that act both locally and throughout the body to increase blood pressure. A vicious circle develops since the higher the blood pressure, the more the kidney gets leaky and doesn't work well. Eventually this can lead to kidney failure.

Factors in the development of kidney disease include:

- genetic factors (family members with either kidney disease or high blood pressure);
- inadequate glucose control;
- high blood pressure;
- inadequate control of blood lipids;
- smoking.

Although renal disease is a serious complication, not all people with diabetes will develop renal problems. Only about one third of people with diabetes are at risk for renal disease. Excellent glucose control improves the chances of never having diabetes-related kidney disease.

When the kidneys no longer work to clean your blood, there is a buildup of substances normally excreted, one of them being "creatinine." Creatinine is formed every day because you make and remake your muscle cells and creatinine is the by-product. Normally it is excreted and you have a stable low level in your blood. One way to measure the degree of kidney failure is to look at the level of creatinine left in the blood. If it is too high you feel very ill. As well, if the kidneys are leaking protein, the most important of these is albumen. Albumen is normally not in the urine but may be found there if changes from diabetes begin to occur in the kidney. Kidney function is checked by:

- measuring the creatinine in the blood and using this to estimate the glomerular filtration rate (eGFR);
- looking for spillage of albumin in the urine by assessing the albumen/creatinine ratio (ACR) in a routine urine test;
- checking the urine for signs of infection or abnormal cells or "casts" (microscopic debris) that may suggest other reasons for kidney problems;
- evaluating a sample of urine collected over 24 hours to determine kidney function and total protein (albumen or other proteins).

Increased loss of protein is an early warning sign of future renal disease. Use of an ACE inhibitor, even without evidence of high blood pressure, has been shown to be helpful. Optimal blood pressure should be under 130/80 to minimize proteinuria and the progression of renal disease.

Once the ability of your kidneys to clear toxic substances has fallen to half of normal, or if significant protein is being lost, it is important that you see a kidney specialist. Various therapies and these should be discussed so both you and the doctor are prepared for either dialysis or transplant long before they are required.

## Dialysis

If the waste products build up too high, they must be "dialyzed" out. "Dialysis" is the term used to describe a system that allows clearing of the waste products—either inside a person's abdomen by putting in and taking out a fluid (peritoneal) or by removing blood from the person and running it against a membrane that allows the waste products to leave (hemodialysis).

## Transplant

People with diabetes actually do well if they receive a kidney transplant. After a transplant you must take medicine to stop your body from rejecting the "foreign" organ. Unfortunately, these medications have side effects since their job is to lower the body's immune system.

An exciting possibility for anyone having a kidney transplant and therefore taking anti-rejection drugs is to do a pancreatic transplant at the same time or after a renal transplant. This allows the body to normalize glucose levels and maintain good kidney function in the new kidney.

There are no signs or symptoms to indicate that you have kidney damage. Thus, it is very important for you to be screened for kidney changes yearly. Yearly screening should start five years after puberty in type 1 diabetes and at diagnosis in type 2 diabetes.

### 3. Neuropathy

"Neuro" means related to the nerves or nervous system, "pathy" means disease or morbid condition.

> James had also told the doctor about the burning in his feet that he was experiencing at night. He tries to sleep with his feet sticking out the side of the bed because the weight of the bedclothes is just too much.

As with any diabetes complication, prevention is the key. People are often diagnosed with type 2 diabetes when they complain about changes in nerve function, such as numbness or pain in their feet, which is one of the most common complications of diabetes, occurring in about 50 percent of those with type 2 diabetes. Neuropathy tends to respond to improved glucose control better than most of the other microvascular complications. All the nerve complications are affected by the level of glucose control. The better your blood glucose levels the less likely you are to develop neuropathy. If you already have neuropathy, improving your blood glucose control can slow its progression. If you have sensory nerve changes, it must be remembered that glucose is not the only thing that will damage nerves and other reasons for changes in sensation must be ruled out. These include such things as vitamin deficiencies (thiamine or $B_{12}$), the excessive use of alcohol, chronic severe infections such as HIV and some tumors.

*What is "sensory polyneuropathy"?*
The sensory nerves take information about touch, temperature, or pressure back to the brain for processing. The most common way that nerves can be affected is by glycosylation (attachment of sugars). This affects the proteins associated with the nerve so the information sent by electrical pulses is slowed or does not happen. This is seen first in the gradual loss of sensation in the longest nerves, those going to the toes. The pattern of loss of sensation is often in a "stocking or glove" distribution, meaning that it covers an area the same as a stocking or glove would.

Sometimes, the sensation is not lost, but distorted so that people complain of burning or throbbing, sharp or stabbing pains. Improving blood glucose management is thought to be the best and first line of treatment for painful neuropathy. Recent studies suggest that the more someone's glucose level fluctuates, the more likely that there will be discomfort. Many medications have been tried for the relief of painful symptoms. Some are more effective than others. Some of the following medications are used to treat diabetic neuropathic symptoms, but their primary use may have been to treat other diseases or conditions. These medications may be used "off label"—a term that means that the doctor prescribes it to treat a condition other than its original approved use.

- Tricyclic antidepressants, such as amitriptyline or imipramine are often tried first. Exactly how these medications help we are not sure, but the side effects, such as feeling tired or sedated, dry mouth, constipation, urinary retention, or postural hypotension (a drop in blood pressure caused by a sudden change of position), sometimes limit their use.

- Anticonvulsant medications, such as gabapentin and car-
  bamazepine are often used for the relief of symptoms.
  More recently, pre-gabalin has shown promise, providing pain relief within a week of starting it at doses of 300
  to 600 mg. Lamotrogine and sodium valproate have also
  been shown to help in some people. The dose often must
  be brought up slowly for these medications, which seems
  to limit side effects. This group of medications may work
  by suppressing the abnormal electrical firing of the
  damaged nerve endings.
- Wearing a patch of a local anaesthetic (lidocaine) can be
  a promising therapy for relieving pain with few side
  effects.
- Other topical creams, such as capsaicin (made from hot
  peppers) might act locally to subdue the local molecules
  that produce pain. Even a locally applied nitroglycerin
  patch can help in relief of localized symptoms.
- Pain treatments, such as opiates (codeine derivatives)
  might be needed for some patients, alone or in combination with other agents.
- Acupuncture has been used and some studies have
  reported pain relief for up to six months. More trials are
  needed to show that acupuncture does work.

Treatment of painful neuropathy continues to be a challenge
as there is no really effective treatment that works for everyone. The best treatments known to control the pain include
attaining the best possible glucose control with the fewest ups
and downs, and finding the medication mix that works best
for you. Anyone with significant neuropathy has a marked
increased risk of foot ulcers. But remember that a foot does
not ulcerate all by itself. In order to provide support for your

feet, it is vital that you wear comfortable, well-fitting footwear and that you care for your feet daily. See Appendix Three for detailed foot care recommendations.

## What is "mononeuritis"?

Mononeuritis is the lack of function of one nerve, which often occurs suddenly due to blockages to the tiny blood vessels that supply oxygen and nutrients to individual nerves. The condition can affect any nerve in the body but some of the more common ones are:

- a nerve may lead to controlling eye movements;
- a nerve to an ear, may lead to deafness in that ear;
- a nerve providing sensation and movement to one side of the face may lead to Bell's palsy;
- a nerve that helps hold the foot up, may lead to a foot drop.

In most cases, excellent glucose control, occasionally a short course of steroid medication. and time (six weeks to six months) will resolve the problem. Sometimes there is permanent loss of nerve function. Very rarely, the same sort of thing can occur relatively quickly in different nerves, often in the shoulder and hip area, and frequently is associated with a degree of mental depression. This is called "mononeuritis multiplex" or "amyotrophic polyneuropathy." When this occurs, excellent glucose control, often a course of steroids, physiotherapy, antidepressants, and a longer period of time are needed to recover. This more extensive neuritis can take from six months to more than a year to get better.

## What is "autonomic" neuropathy?

The nerves most commonly affected by neuropathy are:

- sensory (which provide feelings such as touch, hot, cold);
- motor (which send messages from the brain to the muscles to move).

However, other nerves in the body called autonomic nerves can be affected. These nerves control functions of the body that you normally wouldn't think about, such as how fast the contractions in your gut push the food down, whether you control your blood pressure when you stand up, and whether you have an erection or sense arousal when you have sex.

Constipation is one of the most common problems. This can be helped by eating high-fiber foods, increasing water intake, and exercising. Occasionally, the use of a stool softener or high-fiber medication can help.

Another common problem is erectile dysfunction (impotence). Normal erectile function requires both a good blood supply and functioning nerves. In diabetes, often one or both of these are affected. Medications are available that will often help, particularly if part of the problem is related to blood flow. If the medications do not work, there are other options, such as injections or vacuum-like devices that allow the penis to fill with blood, and there are penile implants.

Rarely, there might be changes in patterns of sweating, so that it happens only on the upper half of the body or while eating (gustatory sweating).

Very rarely, food can travel very quickly through the gut, producing severe and disabling diarrhea. This is often worsened by blood glucose levels bouncing between severe highs and severe lows. When this happens it is important to avoid all hypoglycemia and slowly optimize your glucose control.

On James's next visit to the doctor he mentions that the burning is quite a bit better, no longer does he try to sleep with his feet sticking out the side of the bed. Since going to the diabetes center, James has made some changes to his eating patterns and his blood glucose levels have come down to target level most of the time. James now checks his feet every day and has bought a new pair of golf shoes that fit better and provide good support. He knows that if the burning gets worse or he develops any blisters or problems he should call the doctor sooner rather than later.

*Are my feet at risk of being amputated?*
The combination of decreased sensation and poor blood flow dramatically increases the risk of foot problems. Anyone with decreased sensation has an increased risk of injury to the foot. Infections after injury may occur more easily in the presence of high blood glucose levels. When you have poor circulation to your feet oxygen and protective white blood cells will not easily get to the infected site to help with healing, thus an infection can spread over the foot, into the bone or even into the blood increasing the risk of amputation of the infected area.

The most important preventive measure is for someone with diabetes is to look at their feet regularly to be sure there are no sores or lesions. The presence of *any* sore should be dealt with immediately without delay. You should be sure your doctor looks at your feet; remove your shoes when you go for an examination. Your feet should look like the feet of a baby—no calluses, no cracks, no blisters. Preventive foot care is the best protection. See foot care recommendations in Appendix Three.

## Other Conditions Seen More Frequently in Diabetes

**Depression** has been recognized as occurring more frequently in people with diabetes and it is now known that treatment of depression is likely to help in control of blood glucose. If you feel that you may be experiencing depression, it is important that you discuss this with your doctor, as therapy for the depression will be useful for your overall health (see Chapter Four).

**Non-Alcoholic Steato-Hepatitis (NASH)** We are becoming increasingly aware that some people with diabetes and high blood fats are at much higher risk for a type of liver disease that can lead to liver failure. This is called non-alcoholic steato-hepatitis (NASH) and is a chronic inflammation of the liver cells caused by high fat deposits in the liver. Eventually, the condition can lead to cirrhosis and the need for a liver transplant. As with all complications, good management of blood glucose and blood fat levels reduces the risk.

Complications are a reality in diabetes, but they are not inevitable. Recent studies have shown that complications can be prevented or delayed. Prevention of complications is more than just managing your blood glucose. Blood pressure, blood lipids, healthy nutrition, physical and activity are all important factors to consider in the prevention of complications.

## Screening

Remember not to wait until you have symptoms before you call the doctor! Screening is very important to ensure that treatment, if neces- sary, is started at early stages. The following table outlines the recom- mended frequencies for screening for the different complications.

| Area | Type of Screening | Type of Diabetes | Recommendation |
|---|---|---|---|
| Neuropathy | Assess loss of sensation at great toe. Ask about pain, erectile dys- function, gut symptoms | DM 1 | After 5 years duration once post- pubertal, then annually |
| | | DM 2 | At diagnosis, then annually |
| Retinopathy | Exam by experienced professional | DM 1 | Annually 5 years after onset of diabetes in those ≥ 15 years old |
| | | DM 2 | At time of diagnosis and then every 1–2 years |
| Nephropathy | Random urine ACR and serum creatinine with esitmation of kidney function | DM 1 | After 5 years duration in post- pubertal, then annually |
| | | DM 2 | At diagnosis, then annually |
| Cardiovasular | Resting ECG | DM 1 & 2 | After 15 years duration then every 2 years. At diagnoses if older than 40, or presence of hypertention, protein in urine or reduced pulses, then every 2 years. |
| Dyslipidemia | Fasting lipid profile | DM 1 & 2 | At diagnosis and every 1–3 years LDL-C < 2.0 mmol/L; TC:HDL-C ratio Plasma apo B , 0.9 g/L |
| Hypertension | Take blood pressure | DM 1 & 2 | Measured at every visit, target less than 130/80 |
| Foot care | Examine the foot | DM1 & 2 | Evaluated each visit, especially if any evidence of nerve or blood vessel disease |

Canadian Diabetes Association 2008 *Clinical Practice Guidelines*

# TEN

# *Making Young and Getting Old*

The creation of a family is a significant commitment. Women with diabetes can have families, but there will be some additional factors to consider. Pregnancy is a happy life event although very stressful. The management of the diabetes will produce additional stresses. Therefore, when you plan a pregnancy, it is important to consider your resources and support systems for handling stress.

*Diane's story*
Diane has had diabetes since she was five years old and she has learned to manage her diabetes well. She takes insulin before her meals and at bedtime. She makes daily adjustments to insulin based on the amount of carbohydrate she will eat and her level of activity. Now, she is 27 and has recently married the love of her life, Paul. They have been discussing the possibility of starting a family, but they both want to know more about how Diane's diabetes will affect her pregnancy and their future baby. They also want to know if there is any chance that

Diane's health would be affected by the pregnancy. They go together to discuss these issues with her doctor.

*Yolanda's story*
At 33, Yolanda has been having difficulty getting pregnant because she has always had irregular periods. Her doctor recently told her that she has a disorder called polycystic ovarian disease and, when he did some tests, discovered that she also has type 2 diabetes. Since being told of the diagnosis she has checked her glucose rarely, usually in the morning, the levels are about 7 mmol/L. Her doctor has suggested that she see the dietitian to get a plan for healthy eating and that she begin an exercise routine. He mentioned that she may need to start a medication called metformin or possibly insulin if her glucose did not reach the target levels with a healthy meal plan and exercise.

Both these women have diabetes and are contemplating pregnancy. Some of the issues they need to consider are similar, others are different.

**Can I Get Pregnant If I Have Diabetes?**
Yes, if you have reasonably well-controlled type 1 diabetes, it is unlikely that you will have any more difficulty becoming pregnant than a woman without diabetes. If you have type 2 diabetes, you might have a bit more difficulty getting pregnant. Type 2 diabetes is more often associated with excess weight, especially around the waist. If you have excess weight, there may be a change in your hormone balance. The combination of irregular periods, inconsistent ovulation and possibly the evidence of more male hormone than usual—an effect that

shows up as excess hair (hirsutism)—is often termed "polycystic ovary syndrome." This is seen more often in women with insulin resistance, with or without diabetes. If you have polycystic ovary syndrome, you can improve your chances of ovulating and thus becoming pregnant by reducing your level of insulin resistance. This can be done by adjusting your eating habits to decrease the need for insulin. You can also increase your insulin's effectiveness with regular exercise. Should these measures not work to normalize periods, metformin might be tried in an effort to reduce insulin resistance and help ovulation. Insulin can be and should be initiated prior to pregnancy if the glucose control is not optimal.

**Will My Insulin Requirements Change during Pregnancy?**
Your insulin needs change during pregnancy. There is usually an increase in insulin requirements almost as soon as you know that you are pregnant. Particularly if you have type 1 diabetes, you may have a marked risk of hypoglycemic episodes, predominantly at night in the first trimester, even though your overall insulin needs go up. Nearing the end of the first trimester and in the early second trimester (8 to 14 weeks), there is a mild decrease in the natural insulin resistance during any pregnancy. During this period, the anti-insulin hormones might decrease slightly as the support of the pregnancy shifts from the ovary to the establishing placenta. At this time, the risk of hypoglycemia is often greatest. It is also important to realize that the ability to sense low blood glucose might decrease during pregnancy, which can lead to hypoglycemia unawareness (see Chapter Eight). To protect against unexpected hypoglycemia, you will need to take particular care to check often enough to catch a lowered blood glucose level before it becomes severe.

Once the placenta is established, it produces hormones in progressively greater amounts until almost the end of the pregnancy. Some of these hormones increase insulin resistance, which results in insulin needs being raised to two to three times normal amounts by the end of the pregnancy. In the last one to three weeks of the pregacy, the insulin required may decrease. This happens because the placental growth falls off and it gets "old," with a decrease in the anti-insulin hormones that it produces. The baby also grows quickly as the end of the pregnancy approaches, so the transfer of food (and glucose) to the baby, increases. If insulin requirements fall off too rapidly at the end of pregnancy, this can be a sign of problems with the pregnancy or the placenta.

Women with type 2 diabetes might not be on insulin prior to pregnancy but will likely need insulin during pregnancy to keep their glucose level normal. If you have type 2 diabetes, your ability to make insulin is already decreased. The normal weight gain of the pregnancy and the resistance that increases due to placental hormones means that you will need more insulin. Insulin is the safest treatment, because it does not cross the placenta and is normally present in the mother anyway. If you are on oral medication to manage your diabetes prior to pregnancy, it is often wise to switch to insulin and become comfortable with its adjustment before becoming pregnant.

### What Are the Chances That My Health Will Get Worse during Pregnancy?

Even if you have diabetes, pregnancy—as for most women—is a healthy event. It is unlikely that your health will worsen due to the pregnancy, particularly if you have none of the complications of diabetes. If complications from diabetes are present, you might be at risk for worsening of these during and following the pregnancy. If you have any form of diabetes, before you get pregnant it is important that you are sure that you have no unsuspected complications that might affect the success of your pregnancy or your future health. You and your doctor must be sure that:

- glucose control is optimal;
- you are aware of existing micro/macrovascular complications.

### How Will My Doctor Check for Complications of the Diabetes before Pregnancy?

Looking for any signs of complications prior to pregnancy would include:

1. *An eye examination* (done by a specialist in diabetes eye disease or ophthalmologist) to ensure there is no retinal disease. This eye exam may find:
   - no retinopathy, which means you have very little risk of any changes occurring to your eyes or your vision during pregnancy.
   - background retinal disease or minor changes in the blood vessels from the diabetes, which means there is little risk to your vision if:
     - glucose is well controlled
     - blood pressure is well controlled
     - you see your eye doctor regularly during pregnancy and after to be sure that there are no changes.
   - "proliferative" retinopathy or areas of new vessel formation, in which case there is potential for serious eye changes that could become worse if you get pregnant. Any proliferative changes might worsen if your control is not good and you suddenly improve your glucose levels. In

pregnancy, if your glucose control is anything but excellent, efforts will be made to improve your glucose as quickly as possible, for the safety of the development of the baby. Targets are lower than those expected in women with type 1 who are not pregnant. As well, in a pregnancy there may be increased growth factors, which promote the formation of new vessels. The combined factors of a fast and dramatic lowering of glucose to normal with growth factors in abundance, has been associated with marked worsening of proliferative or pre-proliferative eye disease in early pregnancy. If you do have proliferative eye changes, the best thing to do is to bring your glucose levels as close to normal as you can gradually (over two to four months)before getting pregnant (see Chapter Nine). Your eye specialist may recommend laser treatment to protect your vision. Once treated effectively, the eye changes can be corrected (or remain "quiescent" or quiet) and it may be safe to consider pregnancy without worrying about loss of vision.

## 2. An assessment of kidney function:

- a routine urine test to be sure there is no infection or other abnormality.
- a special urine test to determine if there is any leakage of protein. Usually you will be asked for a routine urine test sent for an albumin/creatinine ratio (See Chapter Nine). If this is abnormal, your doctor might ask for additional tests, such as 24-hour urine for protein, micro-albumin, and creatinine clearance.

In the majority of cases, there are no abnormalities, but if they are found, they indicate the need for significant attention to your glucose and blood pressure control throughout the pregnancy.

Only if you have significant changes in renal function, prior to pregnancy, are there major risks of the progression of renal disease during the pregnancy and potential risks to the fetus. Therefore, if you have any renal disease before you get pregnant, it is very important that your condition is followed in a high-risk pregnancy clinic by a health care team used to dealing with these abnormalities. In a few cases, where there is very poor kidney function before the pregnancy, it can worsen dramatically during pregnancy; therefore, pregnancy may not be advisable for these women.

*3. An assessment of potential cardiovascular risks:*
### Hypertension
If you have hypertension diagnosed before the pregnancy, your risk for blood pressure–related problems will be higher than normal. Some medications commonly used to treat blood pressure in diabetes are not to be taken by a pregnant woman. The most important of these are the angiotensin converting enzyme (ACE) inhibitors and the angiotensin receptor blockers (ARBs). If you are taking either of these types of medication to control blood pressure before a pregnancy, they should be changed to another antihypertensive medication known to be safe during pregnancy *before* you become pregnant.

### High cholesterol or abnormal blood lipids
Medication to improve your blood fats (cholesterol or triglycerides) called "statins" and "fibrates" are not to be taken by pregnant women and should be stopped before pregnancy. If they were not stopped before, they should be stopped as soon as you know that you are pregnant. Rarely would very high blood lipids present a risk in pregnancy. If you have a more significant lipid problem, you should discuss your particular risks with your doctor.

### Hidden heart disease

Your doctor might want you to have an electrocardiogram before pregnancy to be sure that there is no evidence of strain on the heart. If you have had type 2 diabetes for 5 to 10 years or you smoke, particularly if you are older, you could require additional tests to be sure that your heart is working well.

### Why Should My Glucose Control Be Good Before I Get Pregnant?

The majority of women and their babies do well in the presence of diabetes. However, the higher the levels of glucose or A1C before pregnancy, the higher the risk of having a baby with a birth defect (congenital malformation). The chance of a birth defect in any pregnancy is about 1 percent. This risk doubles once the glucose levels are in the range just above those that make the diagnosis of diabetes and increases further if the glucose levels are higher, to about 4 to 7 percent. Remember, this means the chances of the baby being perfectly normal are 93 to 96 percent. To reduce the chances of any problems, it is strongly recommended that women with either type 1 or 2 diabetes who are planning their pregnancy be sure that their glucose control is as normal as they can safely make it. By the time you know that you are pregnant, important major fetal organ formation has already begun, so the improvement of blood glucose levels should be achieved *before* the pregnancy.

You should try to reach glucose control as close to normal glucose control as possible while you are trying to get pregnant, providing it is safe for you to do so. That means, when possible, your A1C is lower than 6 percent, and at least lower than 7 percent. It means your fasting and pre-meal glucose levels should be lower than 5.3 mmol/L (95 mg/dl) if that can be safely achieved (possible in most women with type 2 diabetes) but at least lower than 7 mmol/L (126 mg/dl). Your glucose levels should be lower than 7.8 mmol/L (140 mg/dl) at one hour and lower than 6.7 mmol/L (120 mg/dl) at two hours after the meal, whenever possible. In order to achieve these levels, you have to pay detailed attention to your eating habits and physical activity.

To further reduce the chances of any abnormality, a supplement of 5mg of folic acid should be started 3 months prior to pregnancy through the twelfth week of pregnancy, after which doses of only 0.4–1 mg of folic acid in a multivitamin can be continued until the end of lactation. It has been shown to reduce the risks of fetal neurological abnormalities in pregnant women with health risks such as diabetes.

The normal growth of the fetus is optimal when glucose control is optimal. This is very important in the second trimester as the baby's brain and the islet cells are forming. In the third trimester, if glucose values are elevated, the baby may effectively be "fed" too well, make more than normal of its own insulin and potentially grow bigger and fatter. If this happens, the baby may not be as healthy in utero, so attention is often paid to monitoring the fetus more carefully.

Women with diabetes who are pregnant have been shown to have the best outcomes if they are followed by a health care team experienced in the management of diabetes and pregnancy. If this sort of expertise is available in your area, you should try to arrange an appointment while you are planning your pregnancy. This way, you can ask all your questions and you can be sure that your control is optimal. Establishing (with your team) the diabetes regimen that will be used during pregnancy is important because once you are pregnant, changing the regimen might cause a short-term slip in glucose control at an important time in the baby's development.

**Can I Take Oral Medications While Pregnant?**

Recently, there have been studies done of certain oral medications for diabetes that are used in pregnancy. Of the insulin-releasing medications, only glyburide crosses the placenta minimally and has thus been studied. The immediate pregnancy outcomes appear to be safe compared to those using insulin as long as good glucose control is achieved. As yet, the numbers of women treated in pregnancy in good study trials do not clearly tell us that all pregnancy-related immediate and any long-term risks for the baby are not increased. As yet, glyburide use is not considered to be optimal care in pregnancy.

The insulin sensitizing medication, metformin, has also been used in clinical trials during both conception and pregnancy. The medication might improve the chances of conception and decrease early pregnancy losses in women with significant insulin resistance. This treatment's safety during the pregnancy is the subject of ongoing randomized trials that should help clarify the drug's status. At the present time, it is considered a drug that could be used during pregnancy but that may have unknown effects.

**What Are the Chances That My Child Will Have Diabetes?**

Babies of women with diabetes do not have diabetes at birth. For women with type 1 diabetes, the risk of type 1 in your children is also very rare—1.3 to 4 percent. There are currently studies being done to try to develop genetic testing for these children, to assess their risks. Although there is currently no effective therapy to prevent type 1 diabetes, attempts are being made to identify any "at risk" children, as it is hoped that some therapy might one day be available.

Inadequate glucose control in pregnancy might increase the chance that the baby is born too big (macrosomic). On the other hand, women with type 2 diabetes, particularly if they also have high blood pressure, can have babies that are too small. Children born either too big or too small, of women with either type 1 or type 2 diabetes, have been shown to have an increased future risk for obesity, high blood pressure, abnormal fats in their blood, and/or diabetes when they become adults. The closer to normal the mother's glucose, the less chance the baby's growth in the womb will be affected, likely reducing any further effects on his/her glucose tolerance. Long-term studies are under way to try to determine how great these risks are and which babies are at higher risk. The role of genetic risk has not been made clear, but genetic risks are higher in type 2 than type 1 diabetes.

Breast-feeding helps to protect your child against obesity and to reduce the risk of diabetes. It is important to continue to control your own glucose well while breast-feeding because we know that glucose is transferred in the milk. It is also important to continue to take a multivitamin with 0.4–1 mg of folic acid while breastfeeding.

### What If I Don't Want to Get Pregnant—What Contraception Methods Are Safe?

Most contraception methods that are safe and effective for any woman can be used in women with diabetes. The specific method that is likely to work best for you should be discussed between you and your doctor.

As always, mechanical protection or condoms, if used appropriately, provide protection with the minimum of risk that the method will affect your diabetes. Equally, such usage will mean that any risk of sexually transmitted infections is minimal. However, condoms—as a long-term method of contraception—do not have the best protection rates, mainly due to misuse or non-use at the wrong times.

A low-dose estrogen birth control pill (the pill) is usually an effective contraceptive and, in most cases, affects blood glucose control minimally. You may notice either a slight increase or decrease in insulin requirements, although often the insulin dosages do not change. Similar mild changes in oral medication requirements might be noted if you are on the pill. As with any change, if you start taking the birth control pill you will need to check more frequently and possibly make adjustments to your treatment when you either start or stop taking the pill. Any other risks, such as a tendency to thrombophlebitis or clotting disorders, may mean you cannot take the pill. The use of a contraception using progesterone only, by injection every three months, is felt to add to cardiovascular risk and is not advisable.

You could use an IUD (intra-uterine device), although these devices can cause heavy menstrual bleeding. They are not infallible; rarely conception will occur with an IUD in place. More importantly, with diabetes you might be at a somewhat increased risk for infection of the uterine lining due to the presence of a foreign body. This would be a problem if your glucose control is not good, as your risk of infection might be increased. You must be especially vigilant if you develop a foul-smelling vaginal discharge and, if present, the IUD must be promptly removed and antibiotic treatment begun.

Once your family is complete, a tubal ligation—which blocks the ability of the sperm to reach the eggs released from the ovary—is the safest form of contraception. If a woman is having a caesarean section and plans no more children, this minor operation can be done right after the caesarean and would not require additional anaesthesia or recovery time. If not, there would be some surgical risk if the minor operation (usually day surgery) is done. Since any form of surgery for a woman with diabetes requires special adjustments of diet and therapy, for some couples, a vasectomy done on the male partner might ultimately be safer. Clearly, this needs to be worked out between the couple with advice from their doctors.

**For the Guys ... Should I Have Any Concerns about Having Children?**
Fertility is usually not a problem for a man with diabetes; however, there might be some reduction in your ability to conceive if you are severely overweight or have very poor glucose control. It is important not only to improve on either or both of these problems, but also to remember that a pregnancy is a long-term commitment to remaining healthy to care for the child. The decision to start a family should include a decision to commit to optimizing lifestyle and glucose control on a long-term basis.

The children of men with diabetes also have an increased risk of future diabetes. In fact, if you have type 1 diabetes, and especially if you were young when you became diabetic, your children have a slightly higher risk than if the mother has type 1 diabetes—in the 6 to 9 percent range compared to 1.3 to 4 percent risk for mothers with type 1. Just as for women with type 1, as a man with type 1 diabetes you might want to participate in studies involving genetic testing for your child. If you have type 2 diabetes, the long-term risk of your child developing the condition is increased, although the genetic links have not been clearly identified.

*Erectile dysfunction (ED) or impotence* is the most common problem involving the reproductive system in men with diabetes. This condition will not necessarily affect the ability to conceive a baby; however, it definitely makes it more difficult! The presence of erectile dysfunction in men with diabetes can be due to macrovascular disease (blood flow regulation and availability reduced) or microvascular disease (nerves that control the process of engorgement of the penis do not work properly). In the case of macrovascular causes, it is important to rule out any other kinds of large-vessel disease, such as heart disease. Regardless of whether the ED is caused by macro- or microvascular disease, there are medications that allow improved blood flow and can often help. If you have already tried this unsuccessfully, it is important to see a urologist to be sure there are no other problems and to discuss additional therapies (devices, injections, and penile implants).

## Diabetes in the Older Adult

When does one become an "older" adult? Is it 60, 65, or older? How you define getting older does not really matter; the important thing is to get there and to be as healthy as you can be. Some older adults will have had diabetes for many years and have learned how to manage it along with whatever else arises as they age. Others will develop diabetes in this stage of life. For these people, making adjustments to habits and lifestyle of a lifetime may be very difficult.

*Elizabeth's story*
Elisabeth is 70 years old, she has lived alone since her husband died three years ago. She recently had her checkup at the doctor's office and was told she now has type 2 diabetes. Elisabeth was not surprised; her mother also had diabetes when she was in her 70s. She has been lonely since her husband passed away, and has been thinking that she should get involved with some other older adults. She says that the diagnosis of diabetes is just the impetus she needed to get her down to the community center to sign up.

Anyone who is over 40 who develops diabetes is more likely to have type 2 than type 1, although it is possible to develop type 1 at any age. The condition might go undiagnosed for some time because the symptoms are easily put aside as those of aging. Having less energy, getting up at night to go to the bathroom, deteriorating eyesight, and so on are expected symptoms of aging and might not be thought important enough to discuss with your doctor. As an older adult, you may not have the same symptoms of diabetes as a younger person. Due to the changes associated with aging, you might not feel thirsty, and other symptoms could be masked by other medications you take. Unfortunately, this means that by the time diabetes is diagnosed, you may have had it for many years and some of the complications may be present. It is not uncommon for a person to have a heart attack caused by diabetes before knowing he/she had diabetes.

The diagnostic criteria for diabetes are the same for people of all ages. These are a fasting level of more than 7.0 mmol/L (126 mg/dl) on two occasions and/or a blood glucose at another time of day of at least 11.1 mmol/L (200 mg/dl) on two occasions or the presence of symptoms of diabetes with abnormal glucose (see Chapter Three).

**Will Menopause Change Anything Related to My Diabetes?**
Menopause may be relatively unnoticed, or be associated with significant symptoms. The presence or absence of diabetes does not affect this. Sometimes there is more variation in the glucose levels if there are bigger variations in hormone levels. Some women experience significant hot flushes at menopause. It may be hard to tell whether you are having a nighttime low glucose level, making you feel hot and sweaty, or if you are having a hot flush. The only way to be sure is to check the glucose level.

The advisability of hormone replacement therapy for women

with diabetes has been questioned. Generally speaking, if you have difficult symptoms related to menopause, a short period of hormone replacement might be justified. For the majority of women, this is not the case and the current feeling is to let nature take its course. Opinions on the value of hormone replacement therapy have fluctuated for last 20 years. However, the results of several studies that followed a significant number of women for several years have led the medical community away from its long-term use.

### Does the Management of Diabetes Change in Older People?

The management of diabetes in the older adult is the same as in the younger adult. If you are otherwise healthy, your targets for blood glucose levels, blood pressure, and lipids should be the same as for the general population with diabetes (see Chapter Three). It is important to discuss your target levels with your doctor or health care team, especially if you have any other medical conditions.

### *Nutrition*

How and what you eat is very important, which is why, as an older adult, you should consult a dietitian to develop an individualized healthy meal plan. If you cannot see a dietitian, consider getting one of the cookbooks listed in Resources at the end of the book. Cooking for one can seem more difficult, especially when it comes to planning healthy nutritious meals—there's always a danger that you might lose the motivation to take care of yourself. If you don't like eating by yourself, consider joining a social club, community group, or religious organization to find opportunities for companionship and variety in meals. As you age, your appetite often diminishes; the important thing is to eat regular and balanced meals.

*Changes That Can Affect Your Eating Habits As You Age*
The following are some of the changes that occur with aging
and some suggestions for coping with them.

- Intestinal slowing can mean that you do not absorb the
  nutrients as well or that food absorption is slower. This
  can lead to a tendency to constipation. As for anyone with
  this problem, increasing fiber in your diet will help, such
  as bran cereals, prunes in small amounts, or over-the-
  counter medications that increase fibre. Sometimes a liquid
  nutritional supplement will allow adequate nutrition, and
  maintaining adequate fluid intake can help as well.
- Thirst might be reduced so that you have more risk of
  becoming dehydrated. Sometimes you need to force yourself to drink water, soups, or tea and coffee to get enough
  fluids during the day.
- The ability to make insulin falls off with time, and the release
  may be slower, so large meals would lead to poorer glucose
  control; more frequent small meals might work better.
- You might not have the energy to shop and prepare meals.
  Even things such as chopping foods, stirring the batter,
  or chewing might become increasingly more difficult.
- The state of your teeth has an impact on your ability to
  eat properly and comfortably. If you have dentures that
  do not fit properly, eating will become very difficult and
  you will probably eat less and not enjoy your meals as
  much. Regular dental care is a must.
- If you have difficulty swallowing, there are specialized
  teams at most hospitals to help you overcome this problem.
  As well, eating or drinking food that is a little thicker, (for
  example, thickened soup rather than a water-based soup),
  might be easier. These sorts of problems can occur after

a stroke and make you afraid of choking. However, it is very important to avoid dehydration; drink all the fluids you can.

- If you have cataracts or other eye disease, you might find cooking, shopping, and reading recipes more difficult. Support programs such as Meals on Wheels are there to help.

- If you do not drive, you may find shopping difficult. Some grocery stores will deliver food for a small fee. Otherwise ask your community center if it has a program that takes seniors shopping, or perhaps you could go with a friend or neighbor.

**Is Physical Activity Important at My Age?**
Yes, physical activity is just as important for you, as an older adult, as for anyone else. You are never too old to benefit from physical activity. Staying active, provides many more benefits in addition to lowering your blood glucose levels. Although it is very important to get moving, it is strongly advised that you speak to your doctor before starting a new activity program. Your doctor will want to make sure that you have no unexpected health issues, such as high blood pressure, heart problems, or circulation difficulties, and that your feet feel normal and have no sores or calluses, which might worsen or change. As you might have had diabetes for some time before you knew it, you could have had a heart attack without any pain (a "silent MI"). Knowledge of underlying health problems does not mean that you cannot increase your physical activity, but it will allow you to do it safely, knowing your limitations.

Once you have the go-ahead from the doctor, you need to decide what to do. Starting and sticking to a program of physical activity might not be easy, but the benefits you gain will make it worthwhile. Usually, it is much easier to do something if you do it with someone else. Most communities have seniors' groups that offer many different activities, some for very fit older adults and some for the less fit. Choose the activity that you feel best fits your state and get started. If you have physical limitations, talk to someone at your community center about programs for people with limitations. There are many and you are sure to find one that suits you.

As you start these activities, consider the following points in relation to your diabetes:

- Check your blood glucose before and after the activity to learn the effect.
- Avoid being active at the time that your medication works its best—check with your doctor or pharmacist about when that is.
- Before you change your activity level, be sure that you know (by checking your blood glucose frequently) what symptoms you get if you have low glucose. If you are on medication that can cause hypoglycemia, be sure to carry with you a source of fast-acting glucose in case you need it.
- Buy a good pair of shoes and break them in slowly. Be sure they are not causing reddened areas or blisters on your feet. Aging makes your skin thinner and it may break down more easily.
- Inform your friends that you have diabetes and tell them what to do should you experience hypoglycemia. If you take any medication it is wise to wear a MedicAlert® identification bracelet or necklace.

Start on your new program of activity slowly. If you have not been active in recent years do not expect to be able to do what you could when you were younger. Start with 5 to 10 minutes a day and gradually work up to at least 30 minutes a day. You don't have to do the 30 minutes all at one time; you could do 10 minutes in the morning, 10 minutes after lunch, and 10 minutes in the evening.

Walking is probably the easiest way to get some exercise. If you do not feel safe or are uncomfortable walking outside, walk in a mall or within your house or building. Some malls even have walking programs for older adults. These programs have the added bonus of being supervised and give you the opportunity to meet others who are trying to stay healthy. If you cannot get to the mall and you live in an apartment, another idea is to walk the corridors in the apartment. Walk up one flight of stairs, walk the length of the corridor, walk down two flights, along the hall and back up one flight and you are back where you started. Do that a couple of times a day and you will have improved your physical fitness.

Resistance training or light weight lifting is another type of activity that is important. Such activity has been shown to improve blood glucose levels as well as increase your overall strength. You do not have to go to a gym to do this. You could use simple household objects, such as soup cans. Start by lifting one in each hand a couple of times, then take a break, then repeat it. You should try to work up to eight lifts repeated three times at least three days a week. Lifting straight out in front of you, above your head, from your waist to your shoulders and in other directions will improve the strength of different groups of muscles.

Even if you are in a wheelchair or are unable to move well, you should try to get some physical activity to keep your blood flowing and your muscles strong. Your doctor or a member of your health care team can give you directions that will outline some wheelchair exercises.

> Elisabeth found that the community center had not just one activity program for older adults but several and at all levels of difficulty. As she had not been active for a while she decided to join the "slow walking" group and now goes out with them three mornings a week. She is finding the walk pleasant and afterward enjoys the camaraderie when they all meet for coffee.

### Are There Any Special Considerations about the Level of Glucose Control for the Older Adult?

There is no doubt that hypoglycemia should be avoided as it is known to increase the risk of falling, which can result in disabling injuries. A fall is often the event that limits independent living. Hypoglycemia also increases the chances of confusion, which is another higher risk area already seen with aging. Received or severe hypoglycemic increases the risks for cardiac event. That being said, the targets for your blood glucose levels should be similar to those for anyone with diabetes.

- before meals: between 4 and 7 mmol/L (72–126 mg/dl);
- At two hours after a meal: under 10 mmol/L (180 mg/dl).

You and your doctor should modify these targets to suit your specific needs. But remember, if you set your targets too high, there are greater chances of impaired brain function, more infections, trouble with involuntary urine loss, and lower levels of energy, any one of which can often limit independent activities. If you take several other medications or have other medical conditions, you may want to raise these target levels somewhat. However, it is important to have the best blood glucose control that you can, as the complications of diabetes (discussed in Chapter Nine) also develop in older adults.

### Will My Medicines for Other Conditions Affect My Diabetes Medication/Treatment?

Medications for diabetes in the older adult are the same as those for younger people. However, hypoglycemia can be more frequent when certain medications are used. Fortunately there are forms of such medications that are slower to be absorbed and therefore reduce the risk of hypoglycemia. If you are experiencing hypoglycemia speak to your doctor to see if your medication should be adjusted.

Many older adults are on medications for other conditions. There is very little, if any, interaction between the diabetes medications and other medication. The biggest challenge being on a lot of medications is remembering to take them. If you have problems remembering to take your medication, try using a "doser" or "dosette." This is a small plastic box, available at the pharmacy, that is divided into sections for different times of the day and different days of the week. Some are small enough that they easily fit into a purse or pocket for when you are out.

Many older adults will have to take insulin to keep their blood glucose levels in the target range. Insulin types, use, and actions are the same as those described in Chapter Seven. Pens are sometimes useful if you have difficulty seeing the marks on a syringe or have developed a shake in your hands. With a pen you can count the clicks as you turn the plunger to set the dose and they are easier to use with unsteady hands.

**Do I Need to Worry about Complications?**
The complications of diabetes, as well as the screening and pre-ventive measures described Chapter Nine, are the same for the older adult as for the younger adult.

No matter how old you are, eating healthy food and staying active are the best preventive tools for enjoying your life. Regardless of your age when diagnosed with diabetes, it is always important to keep your blood glucose levels within the target range; doing so will help you feel well and avoid the complications. Being an older adult when you develop diabetes brings with it some challenges, but your doctor and health care team are there to help you live a full and rewarding life.

# ELEVEN

## *The Path Less Trodden ... New Ideas*

Thirty years ago, we didn't have blood glucose meters at home; we had only one or two choices for oral medications; the insulin was impure and left lumps and bumps; and there were no pumps, pancreas transplants, or islet cell transplants. The area of research and development in diabetes and its treatment has come a long way since then.

*Michelle's story*

Michelle has had diabetes since she was a teenager. She had trouble taking her disease seriously and rebelled a lot. For many years, her glucose levels were all over the place. About 15 years ago, when she developed serious hypertension with changes in her eyes, she began to finally take care of her health, and had laser surgery that saved her sight. Eight years ago she started using a pump and finally had control of her glucose, but even with that and great blood pressure control, she eventually needed a kidney transplant. Now, five years after she received her new kidney, she feels much better than before, but her glucose levels are even more erratic! At her hospital, they are now doing pancreas transplants and told her she is a candidate. She went ahead with the operation and now, one month later she can't believe it! No injections, no worrying about the food she eats—it's like she's "normal"! She still has to take a lot of medications that will keep her body from rejecting both the kidney and the pancreas, but she has a newfound release from the daily pressures of her diabetes control.

## What's New?

### Monitoring Methods
A dream for virtually every person with diabetes is to be able to know his/her glucose level without having to prick a finger. So far, this is not a reality, although researchers are working hard to find an alternative to pricking the finger or arm.

*Will we ever have non-invasive glucose monitoring?*
Researchers are looking tirelessly to try to find a way to determine glucose levels without requiring a needle poke. Present areas of research are:

- infrared systems;
- systems that assess glucose in the fluid around the eye by looking into a tiny laser beam;
- ionic systems.

As yet, these alternatives have not been brought to market, so there are still problems with the techniques.

## Oral insulin

As yet, insulin cannot be taken orally mainly because it is a protein and when taken by mouth, it is digested and made inactive like any other protein that we eat. Researchers are trying to find ways by which the insulin can be combined with a "medium" or carrying substance that would protect the insulin molecule from the digestive enzymes—thus allowing it to work as it should. So far, none of these products appear to be ready for prime time.

## Transdermal insulin

Although not well tested yet, there is a prototype delivery system in development that delivers insulin by a "controlled-release" patch. It remains to be seen if this will be a realistic option.

## Are There Any Drugs That Will Help Control Appetite?

The GLP-1 agonists (for example, exenatide), which feed back to the brain to tell the satiety center that you are satiated or satisfied with the food you have eaten, are likely to help with weight loss in those with diabetes. Studies suggest that they may be very useful in type 2 diabetes if oral agents are failing. Possibly they may be as useful as insulin but with a better chance to promote weight loss. It is too early to know exactly how useful, safe, and well tolerated these agents will prove. There are additional GLP-1 agonists in development.

The investigation of cannabinoid 1 receptor blockers (CB1 inhibitors) is interesting. Apparently, the body has another system in the brain (and maybe the gut) that helps with knowing that we have eaten enough. This system relates to "pleasure-seeking" or "hedonistic" behaviors. It seems that there is a common pathway for those things that the human body finds pleasurable—such as eating and sexual activity, and many addictive substances also act via this mechanism. The active component of marijuana (cannabis) was found to activate this system. There are at least two known cannabis receptors. Investigations have indicated that if you block the action of cannabis receptor 1, the brain senses that you are satisfied. In other words, this inhibitor turns off "the munchies." It also appears to have an effect to decrease the pleasure-seeking behavior in those who crave cigarettes. There is associated nausea in the initial month of treatment, so some people do not tolerate it well. Early studies of its use with a stringent diet for weight loss have shown impressive weight-loss effects associated with improvements in blood fats and diabetes. It does appear that if the drug is stopped, the weight loss effect is lost and may well be reversed. The drug, rimonabant, is the first drug to be evaluated clinically. Issues related to increased depressive tendancies have arisen in larger clinical use. At press, this drug is not on the market.

## Can We Get Islet Cells That Work Back into Our Bodies?

### Pancreas Transplants

In many centers in the world, transplantation of parts of or the entire pancreas is a reality. The pancreas transplant, often done with or after a kidney transplant, can remove the need for injected insulin. As with kidney transplants, which have become relatively routine during the last 30 years, the pancreas transplant now has a much higher success rate. Transplants are usually a whole pancreas transplant where the organ is donated by someone who has died. Some centers do a living-related donor transplant, which means that a family member who matches your genetic makeup can donate half of their pancreas. Luckily, the body can function very well with only half a pancreas although the long-term effects of this on the donor are still being evaluated. There are a number of university centers in Canada currently doing pancreas transplants. The long-term risks of immune suppression (infection, potential increased risk of cancer) must be weighed against the value of doing the transplant. Thus, this treatment will usually be reserved for those already needing a kidney transplant or whose quality of life with diabetes is so poor that the risks for immune suppression are justifiable.

**Islet Cell Transplants**
July 2000, saw a breakthrough, called the "Edmonton Protocol," which has allowed successful transplantation of islet cells alone into the livers of people with diabetes. The islets, as individual cells, re-establish a blood supply in the liver and grow there. This has allowed people with type 1 diabetes to either stop or greatly reduce their insulin injections. The procedure has been limited to those with diabetes with so many glucose swings up and down that their life is virtually unlivable. Luckily, there are not too many people who have that much trouble with the management of their diabetes. There is a limitation to the success of the transplant in that it is difficult to "harvest" enough pancreatic islet cells to reverse the diabetes. The islets must be collected and purified from more than one pancreas. Thus two or sometimes three procedures may be needed to effectively "cure" the diabetes and maintain normal glucose levels. Also, over time, there is a gradual failure of the islet cells so that people usually do not remain insulin independent (80 percent at 1 year, but only 10 percent at 5 years). However, even with a small amount of islet cell function, the diabetes is often substantially easier to control than before the patient received

the transplant. As with whole-pancreas transplants, the transplant patient must take anti-rejection drugs for the rest of his/her life with the risks associated with them.

## Encapsulated Islets

Attempts have been made to remove the islet cells from people who have died, or even from animals, and culture them outside the body, to increase the numbers of available islets. The problem is that islet cells, when put in culture dishes in a lab, forget how to sense glucose and how to make insulin. There continues to be research in this area, as this method would substantially increase the possibility that islet cells in larger quantities would be available and could then be reintroduced. Other efforts are being made to take T-stem cells, which have not yet developed specific functions, and coax them, chemically, to become islet cells.

## Medications to Stimulate the Duct Cells of the Pancreas to Become Islets

An enzyme (INGAP—Islet Neogenesis Gene-Associated Protein) has been found in the body that is able to change duct cells in the pancreas. This enzyme, when injected daily for a period of six weeks into laboratory animals, such as dogs, was able to stimulate the transformation of the ordinary duct cells of the dog's pancreas into newly formed, and functional islets— the whole islet with the insulin-producing cells (beta cells), the glucagon-producing cells (alpha), and the other small numbers of cells normally found in the islet. These islet cells went on to produce enough insulin to eliminate the diabetes that the dogs had. In early-phase studies, this enzyme product is now being tried in humans.

## Convincing Other Gut Cells That Sense Glucose to Secrete Insulin

There are studies under way looking at the possibility of "introducing" the insulin gene into a cell already present in our intestine, a "K" cell. This cell senses glucose and releases an incretin called gastric inhibitory peptide, which works to control liver and other pancreas secretion and gut motility (the movement of food through your gastrointestinal system). These cells already sense glucose and are present in the gut where the glucose arrives and is absorbed. At present, the process of introducing the insulin gene into only those cells has successfully controlled glucose in mice where the pancreas was destroyed. It remains to be seen if this is feasible in species closer to humans.

## Can Anything Be Done to Avoid Complications Other Than Control Glucose?

Researchers are constantly investigating how the various mechanisms lead to both micro- and macrovascular complications. A significant area of interest involves looking for ways to block the formation of glycated end products that are often a common denominator for loss of function in microvascular disease. Additional research on the mechanisms and processes involved in the formation of atheroma or the plaques in the large blood vessels should help in understanding how to reduce the development of macrovascular disease.

By the time this book is in print, there could well be new areas or developments that might have major effects. Research in the field of diabetes is moving very quickly. Diabetes research has brought us a long way from the amazing and life-saving discoveries of the Canadian team of Banting-Best-Collip-Macleod who discovered and purified the hormone insulin.

## Table of Drug Names

| Generic name | Brand Names |
|---|---|
| glyburide | Diabeta |
| | Micronase |
| | Glynase |
| | PresTab |
| | Euglucon |
| glimepiride | Amaryl |
| gliclazide | Diamicron |
| | Diamicron MR |
| glipizide | Glucotrol |
| | Glucotrol XL |
| chlorpropamide | Diabenese |
| tolbutamide | Orinase |
| repaglinide | Gluconorm |
| | Prandin |
| nateglinide | Starlix |
| metformin | Glucophage |
| | Glumetza |
| rosiglitazone | Avandia |
| pioglitazone | Actos |
| acarbose | Glucobay |
| | Precose |
| miglitol | Glyset |
| orlistat | Xenical |
| exenatide | Byetta |
| sitagliptin | Januvia |

Note: this is not an exclusive list of brand names.

Please check with your doctor for availability in the U.S. Some drugs will have different names and there are additional drugs available there and not yet in Canada.

# Resources

**Diabetes Associations**

**Canadian Diabetes Association**
1400-522 University Ave.,
Toronto, ON M5G 2R5
1-800-BANTING

**Diabète Québec**
8550 Pie-IX Boulevard, Suite 300
Montreal, QC
H1Z 4G2
1-800-361-3504

**American Diabetes Association**
1701 North Beauregard St.
Alexandria, VA 22311
1-800-806-7801

**Diabetes UK**
McLead House
10 Parkway
London NW1 7AA
UK

## Web Sites

American Diabetes Association www.diabetes.org
American Medical Association www.ama-assn.org/ama/pub/
category/3158.html
Canadian Diabetes Association www.diabetes.ca
Canadian Health Network
www.canadian-health-network.ca
CDC Diabetes Public Health Resource
www.cdc.gov/diabetes
Diabète Québec www.diabete.qc.ca
Diabetes Insight www.diabetic.org.uk
Diabetes UK www.diabetes.org.uk
Health Canada www.hc-sc.gc.ca/dc-ma/diabete/index_e.html
Healthy Eating Is in Store for You
www.healthyeatingisinstore.ca
International Diabetes Federation www.idf.org
Joslin Diabetes Centre www.joslin.harvard.edu
National Diabetes Education Program www.ndep.nih.gov
National Institute Diabetes and Digestive and Kidney
Diseases www.niddk.nih.gov
U.S. Food and Drug Administration
www.fda.gov/diabetes/glucose.html

For information on specific products such as meters, pumps,
insulin, etc., go to the company Web sites.

## Books

Arsham, Gary, MD, PhD, and Ernest Lowe. *Diabetes: A
Guide to Living Well*, 4th Edition. American Diabetes
Association, 2004.
Barrier, Phyllis. *Type 2 Diabetes for Beginners*. American
Diabetes Association, 2005.

Chiasson, J.L., N. Beaulieu, F. Desrochers, et al. *Understand your Diabetes ... and Live a Healthy Life*. Montreal: Rogers Média Publishing & GlobalMedic, 2005.

Rubin, A.L., and I. Blumer. *Diabetes for Canadians for Dummies*. Toronto: John Wiley & Sons, 2004.

**Cookbooks**

American Diabetes Association and the American Heart Association. *The Diabetes and Heart Healthy Cookbook*. Alexandria, VA: American Diabetes Association, 2004.

American Diabetes Association. *Healthy Calendar Diabetic Cooking*. Alexandria, VA: American Diabetes Association. Available to purchase at www.diabetes.org/.

Blair, Louise and Norma McGough. *Quick Cooking for Diabetes*. London: Pyramid Paperbacks, 2005.

Bowling, Stella. *The Everyday Diabetic Cookbook*. Toronto: Key Porter Books, 1997.

British Diabetic Society. *Diabetic Cookbook*. London: Dorling Kindersley, 2000.

Canadian Diabetes Association. *Beyond the Basics: Meal Planning for Healthy Eating, Diabetes Prevention and Management*. Toronto: Canadian Diabetes Association. Available to purchase online at https://orders.diabetes.ca/cda/.

Canadian Diabetes Association. *Choice Cooking*. Toronto: NC Press, 1982.

Geidt, Frances and Bonnie Sanders Polin, PhD. *The Joslin Diabetes Great Chefs Cook Healthy Cookbook*. New York, NY: Simon & Schuster, 2003.

Good, Phyllis Pellman, *Fix-It and Forget-It Diabetic Cookbook: Slow-Cooker Favorites to Include Everyone!*. Intercourse, PA: Good Books, 2005.

Hollands, Marjorie and Margaret Howard. *Choice Menus Presents: Meal Planning for One or Two People.* Toronto: John Wiley & Sons, in cooperation with the Canadian Diabetes Association, 2004.

Lewycka, Marina. *Caring for Someone with Diabetes.* Brecon, Powys, UK: Age Concern Books, 2004.

Lindsay, Anne. *The Light-Hearted Cookbook.* Toronto: Key Porter Books, in cooperation with the Heart and Stroke Foundation of Ontario, 1988.

———. *Lighthearted Everyday Cooking.* Toronto: Macmillan Canada and the Heart and Stroke Foundation of Canada, 1991.

———. *Anne Lindsay's New Light Cooking.* Toronto: Ballantine Books and the Canadian Medical Association, 1998.

———. *Anne Lindsay's Light Kitchen.* Toronto: John Wiley & Sons, 1993.

Sonksen, Peter, Charles Fox, MD and Sue Judd. *Diabetes at Your Fingertips.* London: Class Publishing, 2003.

Walker, Rosemary and Jill Rogers. *Diabetes: A Practical Guide to Managing your Health*, London: DK Publishing in association with the American Diabetes Association, 2005.

Webb, Robin. *Italian Diabetic Meals in 30 Minutes or Less!* Alexandria, VA: American Diabetes Association, 2005.

Younker, Katherine E. *Complete Canadian Diabetes Cookbook.* Robert Rose in cooperation with The Canadian Diabetes Association, 2005.

# Appendix One

## Meaning of Claims

| Regarding Sugar Content | |
| --- | --- |
| **Claim** | **Meaning** |
| Sugar-free<br>Free of sugar<br>Without sugar<br>Contains no sugar<br>No sugar<br>Zero sugar<br>0 sugar<br>Sugarless | Any of these claims on the label means that there is less than 0.5 g of sugar and fewer than 5 calories from sugar in one serving of this product |
| Reduced sugar<br>Sugar-reduced<br>Reduced in sugar<br>Less sugar<br>Lower sugar<br>Lower in sugar | Any of these claims means that the product has been modified to contain at least 25% less sugar, totaling at least 5 g less sugar per serving than it originally did. |
| No added sugar<br>Without added sugar | This claim means that the product has not had sugar or products containing sugar added to it. It may have natural sugar in the product already. |

Sugars Source: Canadian Sugar Institute. Sugars, Carbohydrates, and The New Food Label, 2004.

| Regarding Fat Content | |
| --- | --- |
| Claim | Meaning |
| Low-fat<br>Low in fat<br>Light in fat<br>Lite in fat | Fewer than or equal to 3 grams of fat per serving<br>**and**<br>Fewer than or equal to 15 grams of fat per 100 grams of dry matter. |
| Lower in fat than ...<br>Reduced in fat | At least 25% less fat than the product being compared<br>**and**<br>1.5 grams less fat per serving or more<br>**and**<br>no increase in energy (calories). |
| Fat-free<br>Contains no fat<br>Very low fat<br>Free of fat<br>Ultra low fat | Fewer than 0.5 grams of fat per serving or referenced amount. |
| Light<br>Lite | These terms can be used only if the product meets one of the above definitions. |

Source: Health Canada www.inspection.gc.ca/english/bureau/labeti/guide/6-2-3e.shtml

# *Appendix Two*

*It is essential that you discuss with your doctor a plan for what to do when you are sick, preferably before you might need it. These recommendations are meant only as general guidelines, and may not be the best plan for you.*

**Sick-Day Management for People Using Insulin**

- **Do not stop taking your insulin**—even if vomiting/not eating—insulin requirements often increase with illness.
- **Check blood glucose and blood/urine ketones** often (every two to four hours).
- **Keep drinking fluids** and, if you are not able to eat, try to take liquids with some sugar and some salt. Here are some examples of fluids with 15 to 20 g of glucose that are easy to sip on if you are ill:
  - 1 cup of juice (taken over an hour). Apple juice (as is or diluted with water) is easily tolerated.
  - 1/2 to 3/4 cup of regular soft drink (taken over an hour), for example, "flat" ginger ale.
  - 1 cup of liquids with some sugar and salt, particularly if vomiting or diarrhea is a problem (for example, soups, Pedialyte, Gatorade, rice water with salt in it).

- **If your blood glucose levels are low** and you have ketones, increase sugar-containing liquids.
- **If your blood glucose levels are high** and you have ketones, add additional rapid-acting or regular insulin every two to six hours with meal (and with snacks if necessary).

*Working with your doctor, fill in the amounts you would need in the chart below:*
Continue your usual intermediate- or long-acting insulin although the dose may need to be decreased if you have low blood glucose.

**My Insulin Adjustment Scale**

My total daily dose of insulin is: _____ units
- 5% of dose is: _____ units
- 10% of dose is: _____ units
- 15% of dose is: _____ units
- 20% of dose is: _____ units

Your doctor should fill in your "usual doses" as well as your actual amount to adjust in units once the calculation of your percentage of Total Daily Dose (TDD) is done.

This table is meant to be a basis or template to help you and your doctor develop a plan in case you become ill. It is only to be used with the help and agreement of your doctor! He or she may have an alternative plan which they would give you.

## Insulin Dose with Adjustments for Illness.

| Usual Dose or Recommended Doses | Breakfast or 0600 | Lunch or 1200 | Supper or 1800 | Bedtime or 2400 | % to adjust |
|---|---|---|---|---|---|
| Intermediate Insulin | | | | | |
| Regular Insulin | | | | | |
| Rapid-acting Insulin | | | | | |
| **Usual dose TDD =** | | | | | |
| Insulin to adjust before each meal: | | | | | |
| ≤ 4 (70) | Treat for low blood glucose and decrease amount by 20 % | | | | |
| 4.1–6.0 (70–110) | __ Usual dose—no change or __ Reduce by 10% | | | | |
| 6.1–10.0 (110–180) | | | | | + 5 % |
| 10.1–12.0 (180–215) | | | | | + 10 % |
| 12.1–14.0 (215–250) | | | | | + 15 % |
| 14.1–18.0 (250–325) | | | | | + 20 % |
| 18.0 (≥ 325) | | | | | + 25 % |

If you are very ill and the insulin adjustment by "sliding scale" seems to have little effect, you may need to apply the increases in the dose every four to six hours if using regular insulin (Novolin ge Toronto, Humulin R) or every three to four hours if you are using a rapid-acting insulin (Novorapid, Humalog).

*Do not hesitate to seek medical help if you are unsure or are not getting better over four to eight hours or ketones are high and you feel ill!*

# *Appendix Three*

*The information about foot care is primarily directed
to people who have evidence of either poor blood flow
or poor sensation in their feet. Hopefully, this will not
be until diabetes has been present for 5 to 10 years at
least. For some people with type 2 diabetes, this may
be the case at the time the diagnosis is actually made.
It is wise for everyone with diabetes to learn the best
way to care for their feet.*

**Basic Foot Care**
- Wash your feet and lower legs daily in warm (not hot) 100°F (37°C) water, with a soft facecloth and mild soap. *Do not* soak your feet.
- Before washing your feet, check them carefully for cuts, bruises, skin breakdown, blisters, or infection. If you cannot see or reach your feet, ask someone to help you or put a mirror on the floor. Be aware of the color of your legs and feet. If you see an injury, swelling, redness, ulceration, or discoloration or have pain, consult your doctor, podiatrist/chiropodist, or nurse specialized in foot care immediately.

- Dry your feet well; be sure to dry between your toes but do not push the toes apart.
- Apply a good skin lotion to heels and soles, dabbing off the excess. Do not apply cream between the toes.
- If you have heel cracks, apply urea cream liberally to heel cracks, cover with plastic wrap and wear loose bed socks overnight, repeating the process until the cracks are healed.
- Bed socks can be worn if they are loose.
- Never wrap anything tightly around your toes.
- People with diabetes are prone to fungus infections (athlete's foot) so you must keep your feet clean and dry at all times. A plain talcum powder or cornstarch can be used daily.
- Never use a cream or ointment on an open wound without consulting your doctor or podiatrist/chiropodist.

### Nail Care

- Cut your toenails in good light, after a bath, when the nails are soft. Use nail clippers or nail scissors but never a knife or rough file. *Do not* peel or pull back nails.
- Cut your nails straight across or in contour to the end of your toe but never down into the corners or below the end of your toes.
- If you have difficulty, consult a podiatrist/chiropodist or nurse specialized in foot care.

### Corns and Calluses

- Corns and calluses are usually caused by pressure from

shoes that do not fit well. They should be treated by a podiatrist/chiropodist or a nurse specially trained in foot care.

- Never cut your own corns or calluses, and do not let a well-meaning friend do it for you.
- Corn cures, plasters, or liquid sold in the pharmacy contain an acid and may burn healthy skin as well as the corn or callus. They should never be used by people with diabetes.

## Shoes and Slippers

- Do not walk barefoot. If you get up during the night, turn on the light and wear slippers.
- Wear good supportive shoes. Supportive shoes are those that:
  - tie up or have velcro closing;
  - come up to the mid foot;
  - have a toe box that is deep enough to allow you to wiggle your toes;
  - are made of a material strong enough to support your foot.
- Always check inside your shoes before putting them on to be sure nothing has fallen in them.
- Check the inside of your shoes for rough spots caused by stitches, seams, or nails as they can cause injury.
- A shoe that is too big is as bad as one that is too small; shoes *must fit* properly.

## Hose/Socks/Stockings

- Always wear the correct size and avoid large seams. If a seam is large, wear the hose inside out. It is possible to buy socks that have no seams.

- Never use garters, elastics, or socks that are tight at the top. These will cut off the circulation and you feet will swell.
- Wear a clean pair daily.
- Choose natural-mix fibers as much as possible as they breathe better.

## Heat and Cold

- Always test the temperature of the water before stepping into the bath; hot water can burn.
- Hot water bottles and electric heating pads can also burn and you may not feel it if you have lost some sensation in your feet. Do not use them.
- Avoid sunburn; use a high SPF lotion or cover up when in the sun.

## Poor Circulation

- *Do not smoke* cigarettes, cigars, or a pipe, or chew tobacco. Inhaling or not inhaling makes no difference. Nicotine constricts the blood vessels and reduces the circulation to your legs.
- Do not sit with your legs crossed or stand for long periods without moving around. Activity keeps your blood circulating.

If you have a cut or scratch, clean the area well with a mild soap and water, and cover with a dry dressing. To clean the area with an antiseptic wash, wash the area with the solution and then cover it with a dry dressing. You can make your own antiseptic wash by mixing 1 tsp (5 mL) of white vinegar in 2 cups (250 mL) of cold water. Mix together in a clean jar and keep no longer than a week.

# Glossary

A1C—glycosylated hemoglobin or hemoglobin A1C—a way to measure the average blood glucose over the past three months by determining the percentage of the hemoglobin molecules in red blood cells that have glucose attached or are glycosylated

Acanthosis nigricans—area of darkened skin at back of neck and under the arms

Adipocytes—fat cells

Adrenergic—symptoms related to the release of adrenalin

Aerobic exercise—exercise that requires increased oxygen for the active muscles

Albuminurea—presence of protein in the urine; small amounts, microalbuminurea, may be a sign of early nephropathy

Anaerobic exercise—exercise that uses fuels that do not require oxygen

Appetite centers—centers in the brain that make you desire food

Atherosclerosis—a global term for blood vessels that have been narrowed or blocked

Autoimmune disorder—when the body mistakenly fights off its own tissues; in type 1 diabetes the body attacks the beta cells

Beta cells—the specialized cells in the Islets of Langerhans that produce insulin

Carbohydrates—the chemical name for molecules that become glucose

Chiropodist—a health care professional trained to treat problems of the feet

Cholesterol—molecules used in the body to make many hormones and carry fats in the blood

Counterregulatory hormones—hormones that are released in

response to falling blood glucose to provide the body with extra glucose

Diabetologist—a doctor who specializes in diabetes care

Diabetes nurse educator—a nurse who specializes in the education and care of people with diabetes

Diabetes education center—a site, usually located in or near a hospital, where a team of health care professionals work together to educate and/or care for people with diabetes

Dietitian—professionals who have at least a bachelor's degree and a year of practical training to advise on diet food and nutrition. "Registered dietitian," "professional dietitian," dietitian are terms protected by law in Canada and can be used only by those with the required training.

Endocrinologist—a doctor who specializes in diseases of the endocrine system, including diabetes

Enzyme—a complex organic compound secreted by cells that produces some form of change

Free fatty acids—break down products of fat cells that can be transported in the blood and used as fuel if needed

Genetic predisposition—chances of inheriting something are greater if it is passed down in the genes

Gestational diabetes—diabetes that first develops during pregnancy

Glucagon—a hormone produced by specialized cells in the Islets of Langerhans that increases blood glucose by stimulating the liver to release glucose

Glucose—a form of sugar used by the cells to make energy

Glycemic index—an index developed to rank foods by how fast and how high the carbohydrate causes the blood glucose to rise

Glycogen—a substance made from sugar that is stored in the liver and muscle. It can be changed back to glucose when needed.

Hyperglycemia—high blood glucose

Hypertension—high blood pressure

Hypoglycemia—low blood glucose, usually defined as below 4 mmol/L (72 mg/dl)

Hypothalamus—a part of the brain that regulates body temperature, appetite, thirst, pleasure-seeking behaviors, and many other processes involved in basic body needs

Hormone—a substance in the body that helps to promote or regulate body functions

Immune system—a complex system in the body that defends against dangerous invaders such as bacteria and viruses or the body's own cells that may have become uncontrolled and will become tumors; a safeguard and cleanup system

Insulin—a hormone produced by beta cells in the Islets of Langerhans that is essential for the metabolism of glucose

Insulin receptors—areas on the cells of the body to which insulin attaches when allowing glucose into the cell

Insulin resistance—a term describing when the body's cells do not respond well to insulin

Internist—a physician who specializes in diagnosis and non-surgical treatments of complex diseases of internal organs

Islets of Langerhans—groups of specialized cells in the pancreas that produce hormones such as insulin, glucagon, somatostatin, and amylin

Lipids—fats in the blood, which include cholesterol and triglycerides

Macrovascular—to do with the large blood vessels

Metabolic syndrome—a cluster of abnormalities that indicate high risk of diabetes and cardiovascular disease

Microvascular—to do with small blood vessels

Nephropathy—kidney damage that may occur due to diabetes

Neuroglycopenic—word for symptoms that occur when the brain does not get enough glucose

Neuropathy—nerve damage that may occur due to diabetes

Nutritionist—a term that is used by anyone wishing to advise on food, diet, and nutrition. The term does not signify any specific training.

Ophthalmologist—doctor who specializes in the diagnosis and treatment of eye diseas; can perform surgery and prescribe medication if needed

Optometrist—specially trained person who evaluates vision and eye health; prescribes glasses if needed

Oral glucose tolerance test—a test to determine if a person has diabetes, blood tests are taken before and after a measured glucose drink

Pancreas—the organ in which the Islets of Langerhans lie and that also secretes many digestive enzymes

Peripheral vascular disease—damage or disease of the blood vessels to the periphery (arms and legs)

Podiatrist—a health care professional trained to treat problems of the feet

Retina—on the back of the eye, senses light; contains many small blood vessels that may become damaged after many years of diabetes

Retinopathy—damage to the eye that may occur due to diabetes

Satiety—the sensation of fullness after eating

Type 1 diabetes—diabetes caused by the destruction of the beta cells; hence the person is unable to make insulin

Type 2 diabetes—diabetes caused by a combination of increasing resistance of the body's cells to insulin and decreasing amounts of available insulin

# Index

Note: A page number in italic indicates an illustration or sidebar.

with type 1 diabetes, 18
with type 2 diabetes, 19
chills, 185
chlorpropamide, 99, *100*
cholesterol
  elevated levels in metabolic syndrome,
    10, *11*
  examination before pregnancy, 226
  HDL, 36–37
  and heart disease, 192
  LDL, 36–37
  and need for insulin, 27
  target levels, 36–37, *38*
circulatory system, 1, *92–93*
claudication, 191
clopidogrel, 201
clots, 179, 194–96
constipation, 216
continuous glucose monitoring systems,
  84–85
contraception, 230–32
corns and calluses, 186, 261–62
corticosteroids, 21
cortisol, 147, 156
cortisone, 8–9, 21, 35, 152, 156
Cushing's disease, 21
cuts on feet, 149
cyclamate, 66

dairy products *see* milk and alternatives
dancing, 70
deafness, 215
delta cells, 5, *6*
denial, 41–42
depression, 43, 218
"designer" insulins, 120–21
detemir insulin, 120, *121*, *127*, 138
Diabète Québec
  contact information, 251, 252
  support groups, 44
Diabetes Education Centres, 51
diabetes mellitus
  benefits, 49
  causes, 20–22
  complications
    about, 188–90
    brain diseases/strokes, 191, 193–94
    depression, 43, 218
    dyslipidemia, *219*

foot problems, 148–49, 194, 217,
  *219*
heart diseases, 190–93, *219*
HHS, 153–54
hypertension, *219*
infections, 146–49
in older adults, 242
ketoacidosis, 149–53
leg problems, 28, 179, 191, 194
macrovascular, 190–201
microvascular, 202–17
nephropathy, 208–12, *219*
neuropathy, 212–17, *219*
non-alcoholic steato-hepatitis, 218
and pregnancy, 224–27
preventing, 196–201
retinopathy, 28, 204–8, *219*
cost to individual and society, 16
definition, 14
diagnosis, 28–29, *31*
famous people with, 14
feelings about, 40–44
gestational, 15, 20–21, 88
and illness, 9, 75, 88, 182–85, 257–59
in children, 18–19, 67, 75
in history, 14
in older adults, 75, 233–42
managing *see main heading* management
prediabetes, *11*, 16–17, 30–31
and pregnancy *see main heading* pregnancy
prevalence, 15
research *see main heading* research
risk factors, 10
supports, 44, 48, 50–51, 125
symptoms, 26
treatment *see main heading* management
type 1
  adjusting for glucose patterns, 171–74
  benefits of physical activity, 68
  definition and causes, 17–18, 22
  proportion of people with, 15
  treatment *see main heading* management
type 2
  adjusting for glucose patterns,
    174–76

272  *Diabetes in Adults*

family and friends
  feelings of guilt, 42
  impact of diagnosis, 40
  supportive role, 44, 48
fasting, 28, 179–82
fat cells
  and amount of insulin needed, 9
  and cholesterol, 199
  and drugs to reduce insulin resistance,
    94
  effects of diabetes drugs, *95*
  and hunger recognition, 8, 12, 93
  in HHS, 153
  in ketoacidosis, 150–51
  in type 2 diabetes, *93*, 94
  and role of insulin, 27
  roles, 8, 92–93
fatigue, 24–26
fats (dietary)
  appropriate amounts, 54–55, 63
  insulin's role in using, 4
  monounsaturated vs. saturated or
    trans, 54, 63–64, 200
  role, 2
  serving size, 60
fats (in blood) *see* lipids
feelings
  acceptance, 44
  anger, 42
  bargaining, 42–43
  denial, 41–42
  depression, 43
  guilt, 42–43
  and physical activity, 67–68
feet
  basic care, 260–61
  blisters, 149
  circulation, 267
  corns and calluses, 261–62
  cuts and scratches, 267
  heat and cold, 267
  nail care, 261
  and neuropathy, 215
  and physical activity, 70–71
  problems, 148–49, 194
  risk of amputation, 92, 194, 217
  shoes, slippers, socks, 70–71, 262–63
fever, 184, 185

fiber, 200
fibrates, 199, 226
flour *see* grains; starches
folic acid, 228
food, *see also* meals
  components and roles, 2
  consulting a dietitian, 50–51
  digestive breakdown
    normal, 1, 3, 6
    with insufficient insulin, 25
  for older adults, 235–37
  healthy eating
    carbohydrates, 59–63
    fats, 63–64
    fruits, vegetables, whole grains,
      53–54
    goals, 51
    lower-fat foods, 54–55
    meal planning, 56, *57*, 164–65
    meal spacing, 52–53
    packaged products, *65–66*, 65
    salt and alcohol, 55–56, 98, 169–71
    serving sizes, 58–59
    sweeteners, 66–67
    to prevent or delay diabetes onset,
      10, *11*
    to prevent heart disease, 200
    variety, 51–52
food labels
  fat content, 256
  sugar content, 255
  understanding, *65–66*, 65, 255–56
fruits
  absorption rate, 53–54
  appropriate amounts, *57*, 200
  carbohydrate content, 60, *61*
  importance of variety, 51
  serving size, 58
fungal infections, 148

gabapentin, 214
gas, 97, 98
gender factors
  alcohol intake, 56
  carbohydrate needs, 61
  diabetes, 15
  heart disease, 191–92
  insulin resistance, 9